Physical Fitness
and
Dynamic Health

THOMAS KIRK CURETON, JR.

Physical Fitness
and
Dynamic Health

THE DIAL PRESS / 1965

DEDICATION

To my wife, Portia Brownell Miller Cureton, who has constantly inspired me to carry on in this work, and to my sons, Kirk Jeffreys and Richard Dozier Cureton

CONTENTS

Part 2 A Practical Program for Physical Fitness

Preface

George Bernard Shaw once observed that "Youth is wasted on the young." One of the many senses in which this statement is so true is that people don't realize what good health means until they've lost it.

Good health is one of life's greatest gifts, but it cannot be taken for granted. Middle age and declining vigor do not occur according to some cosmic timetable; they come when they are invited. All too many of us extend the invitation far too soon.

In the age of the machine when life has become convenient beyond our wildest dreams, when physical exertion threatens to become obsolete, most of us pay more attention to our machines—our cars, our television sets, our dishwashers and our electric shoe polishers—than we do to the condition of our own bodies. Yet our bodies are far more beautiful and complex machines than any man has yet designed or is likely to for a long time.

But unlike man-made machines the human mechanism comes without a set of neatly printed directions on care and use. This is probably fortunate, except that most of us treat our bodies as if they needed no care whatsoever.

This book is a set of directions on the care and maintenance of the human body. It has been prepared by a man who has spent his whole life learning things about the human mechanism that the average person would not suspect. The author, Thomas Kirk Cureton, Jr., has studied the human body at the Physical Fitness Research Center at the University of Illinois, of which he is director. He has tested and trained thousands upon thousands of men and women, young and old, physically fit and out of shape. He has lent his know-how to the Armed Forces, the United States

Olympic Committee, the President's Council on Physical Fitness and countless other organizations.

Into this book he has condensed a lifetime of experience with the character and capacity, the durability and weakness of the human body.

In Part One he explains exactly what physical fitness really means; he offers a method by which you can determine what kind of shape you are in; and he presents a practical exercise program for men and women to regain physical fitness they have lost or hold on to what they have.

In Part Two Dr. Cureton presents a complete twenty-two-lesson course in developing fitness—a course which has been developed over years of work and which is taught in many YMCAs and fitness centers throughout the country. The course involves all the principal muscles of the body in a thoroughgoing and systematic manner. By devoting time to it, anyone can keep his body youthful and thus increase his powers and live more fully the life that is his.

The principles he sets forth have long been in operation at the Physical Fitness Research Center at the University of Illinois. They have been tried and tested for years and have been found beneficial for thousands of men and women.

What Dr. Cureton reveals will surprise many people. First, the most important aim of his program is not to build "muscle men." Instead it is to develop internal fitness—to build up the circulatory system, to exercise the heart and blood vessels, to promote general bodily health on sound scientific principles.

Finally, Dr. Cureton believes that, contrary to what George Bernard Shaw observed, youth need not be wasted on the young. Over the years he has found that no one is too old to undertake his program and, by dint of hard work which won't hurt him in the slightest, regain the peak of trim.

Perhaps the best illustration of what Dr. Cureton has discovered is a story he likes to tell: "In 1948, I was testing some Olympic hopefuls at the Urbana Physical Fitness Center when I noticed a man standing in a doorway over in front of a treadmill. When I got a free moment I approached the man and asked him if I could do anything for him.

" 'Yes,' the stranger replied. 'I have heard about your work and I have come a long way to take your most difficult endurance test on the treadmill.'

"I guessed he was referring to a test in which we run a man on a treadmill to the point of exhaustion and then estimate the amount of blood that has passed through his heart and his lungs. I asked him if he was referring to that test.

" 'Yes,' he said. 'I want to take that test.'

"I took a close look at him and estimated him to be fifty or older. I asked him how old he was.

" 'I am sixty-six now,' he said, 'but I have been training a year and I know I can do well on your test. I have come a long way, so you must give me the test as soon as possible.'

"All my protests and arguments were to no avail, so I finally gave in and told him to change his clothes. Barefooted and clad in only his under-shorts, he mounted the treadmill and proceeded to better the score of ninety per cent of the people we had previously tested on the treadmill.

"Quite amazed at his performance, we questioned him further and learned that he was Lauri Pihkala, a former professor of philosophy who had retired a year earlier from the faculty of the University of Helsinki. On his own, he had developed a method of training in which he alternated steady running and walking at a faster and faster pace over a period of many months. Using this method, he had taken a Finnish runner who thought he had reached his peak and trained him with his new method. Posterity will remember the name of his protégé for a long time, for his runner was the great Paavo Nurmi.

"Now the professor had decided to try the same method on himself, in order to prove to the world that it would work on older men as well.

"Six years later I received a letter containing a newspaper clipping which told how a seventy-two-year-old man had won a twenty-seven-mile open-class cross-country ski race. The winner was none other than my friend Lauri Pihkala. He had dramatically succeeded in his mission."

You will find that both the system and spirit of the old Finn are contained in this book.

THE EDITORS

Physical Fitness
and
Dynamic Health

PART 1

The Meaning
of
Physical Fitness

Section I

WHAT

PHYSICAL FITNESS

MEANS TO YOU

1. Your Life Is in Danger

THE DECLINE OF AMERICA'S FITNESS.   America is rapidly becoming a nation of soft, out-of-shape men and women who cannot endure for an hour the kind of stress that our ancestors faced daily. Today, the typical American is older physically than his years give him the right to be.

The average young man in this country has a middle-aged body. He can't run the length of one city block, he can't swim a hundred yards, he can't climb one flight of stairs without getting out of breath. At the age of twenty-six he has the capacity of a man in his forties. By the time he reaches his early thirties he will have disabilities that are normally associated with men twice his age.

The average middle-aged man in this country is close to death. He is only one emotional shock or one sudden exertion away from a serious heart attack—this nation's leading cause of death.

21

The problem of physical fitness in the United States has grown so serious that the government has felt it necessary to take action and set up the President's Council on Physical Fitness. Gimmicky weight-reducing devices and easy exercise programs have proliferated. We are accused of being a nation of spectators—with justification.

THE THREAT TO THE NATION.   Our lack of physical fitness hurts us nationally. The fact that the rate of rejections from the Armed Forces on physical grounds is appallingly high threatens our national security and indicates a dangerous trend. Certainly it is a cause for thought that the United States Army had to halt the induction of men over thirty-eight primarily because of loss of resiliency, poor resistance to outdoor weather conditions and inability to recuperate from work.

THE THREAT TO YOU.   But much more important than the harm done on the national level is the personal injury that physical unfitness can cause the individual. In all cases it is harmful; in many cases it is actually dangerous.

Being in less than top-notch physical shape prevents us from enjoying life completely because lack of fitness keeps our bodies from operating at peak efficiency. People who can't operate efficiently can't possibly experience and enjoy the infinite pleasure that life has to offer.

More seriously, physical decline involves deterioration of the circulatory system, and inadequate circulation of the blood prevents vital food elements from being distributed sufficiently throughout the body. As a consequence, we are likely to experience a state of fatigue, evidenced by poor posture, awkward movements and low endurance.

Finally and most seriously, lack of physical fitness is a serious health hazard. By getting out of shape we become susceptible to minor ailments, which in turn are the precursors of serious illness. The sobering fact is that the probability of early death is high for seven out of ten people who show a poor fitness picture at the age of twenty-five.

Take a moment to consider how many people you know of who could comfortably experience sudden major physical exertion, besides the athletes you watch on television. You probably can't think of too many. Unfortunately, this situation prevails throughout the country.

LACK OF EXERCISE.   Why does this unhealthy state of affairs exist? Very simply, because people in this country—young people and old people—don't get enough exercise.

Genuine vitality and the zeal of youth come from good circulation of the blood, strong coordinated muscles, and resistance to fatigue and chronic ailments. These desirable qualities can come only from vigorous physical activity.

Modern society is steadily drifting away from the habit of hard work. In an age when man's ability to think is far more valuable than his capacity for physical work, more and more people spend their working hours in a sedentary position. The tasks of daily living are being made steadily easier by an increasing flood of new and ingenious appliances. Thanks to the multiplicity of machines, much of our leisure time is spent in a relaxed position. Instead of walking, we rely on the automobile to carry us to our destination. Thanks to movies, radio, television, professional sports and the like, we have become a nation of sitters and watchers, instead of participants.

We even have machines that are supposed to exercise for us —shaking chairs, vibrating couches and electrical massages; pills, salts and patent medicines—anything to make life easier.

Consider by comparison the daily life of our pioneer forefathers. Without the so-called conveniences of modern living, they had no need for physical fitness programs. For the average man physical activity was part of his way of life. To earn a living, he had to do physical work. To get anywhere, he had to walk, ride a horse, or drive a wagon. To have shelter he had to build a house. With few exceptions, it was probably impossible for anyone to get through a day on the frontier without exerting himself more than the average man does today in a week.

THE UNFAVORABLE EVIDENCE.   The foregoing somber description of the plight of today's Americans is not just constructed from hearsay and a pessimistic frame of mind. It is based on conclusions that I and my associates at the University of Illinois Physical

Fitness Center have reached after two decades of testing thousands of men and women from all walks of life.

We have tested and examined men in various degrees of physical fitness ranging all the way from such outstanding athletes as Roger Bannister to middle-aged, out-of-condition businessmen. The difference in test results between the two extremes is, as you might imagine, wide; even a sedentary worker in good condition is bound to lack the physical capacity of a great athlete.

But the test results provided evidence of a dramatic difference between the people beyond the age of twenty-six who had kept up some sort of exercise program and those who had not. The difference could be measured in a variety of ways: breathing efficiency, heart action, muscular flexibility, circulation, strength and endurance.

I have also seen in my own family the results of physical decline through lack of exercise. My father, a sedentary worker, died far too young, at the age of fifty-eight. By contrast, my mother at eighty-seven still takes a daily swim in the ocean.

Going through my files, I find the following typical example: An athletic coach was the only one out of sixty-five instructors in a war-time program of physical training who failed in several endurance tests. He was told that his failure indicated a poor cardiovascular condition. He had once been a fine athlete, but he had given up training for ten years or more, smoked heavily and indulged himself in rich foods. After he received his diagnosis he refused to do endurance exercises and reduce his weight. Five years after taking his tests he died suddenly—at the age of forty-one.

I could continue through my files and repeat this story many times with only slight variations. Suffice it to say that I have been so impressed by the importance of physical fitness that I have made it my life's work.

THE TREND CAN BE REVERSED.   It has turned out to be a most gratifying occupation, because it has been possible to accomplish a great deal. As I hope to explain in the following pages, I have learned that it is possible for anyone, at any age, to undo damage that may have been done through neglect. It is possible to regain the sort of physical condition that makes life fully worth living.

Furthermore, not only is it in our power to earn "more life for our years," as the expression goes, it is even possible to gain more years for our life. Some authorities believe it possible to add ten to fifteen years to the average life expectancy. Others calculate that the average life span may be increased to 120 years, and the maximum, 150 to 160 years, in contrast to the seventy-two years that is now estimated from actuarial data.

Of course, part of this increase in estimated life span will be the result of a greater survival rate among infants and a greater knowledge of health during middle and old age. As a matter of fact, mankind has already begun to reap these benefits of medical research.

But another part of this increase will come about only if people will learn to and be willing to keep themselves physically fit throughout all the years of their lives. We have found that it is possible for any normal individual to accomplish this—if he goes about exercising the right way.

That is why this book was written, to help you achieve physical fitness—and to hold on to it—by learning how to exercise. It is written, moreover, not on one man's say-so, but as the result of my experience as Director of the Physical Fitness Research Center at the University of Illinois, after testing 20,000 "middle-aged" men from a dozen or more professions and trades. About 3,000 of those who were found able, and were willing to work on themselves, were put through a physical build-up course, and then retested for signs of improved breathing, heart action, muscular flexibility, circulation, strength and endurance.

The general improvement was dramatic, but one conclusion was particularly notable: Cardiovascular ailments among the middle-aged would be negligible if such people would exercise more and eat right.

What we have been able to do for others, in the laboratory, anyone can do for himself, at home. But the first thing you have to do is face the fact that there are no shortcuts to health. There are no "dynamic wonder courses" which will build you up in a short time.

It will take at least three months of hard work—perhaps the hardest work of your life—before you see any significant change. So, before you start on this program, you must really want to improve your physical fitness. In order to do so, you must understand exactly what physical fitness means. You must understand some things about the way your body works. You must be motivated to work as if your life depended on it, for in a very real sense it does.

2. *Physical Decline Means Broken Health*

FITNESS GOES DEEPER THAN APPEARANCE.   It is a characteristic of people in America to approach the problem of physical fitness from the outside in—and never to go farther than skin-deep. The typical person would be happy to have a slim waistline and a good sun tan, and let it go at that.

No one will deny that a good figure and an attractive complexion are desirable. But they are important, not because they contribute to an attractive appearance, but because they reflect an internal well-being that is far more important.

Conversely, the person who allows his physical condition to deteriorate robs himself of more than an attractive appearance. He actually endangers his health.

The most widespread result of premature aging—another way of describing physical deterioration—is the onset of a state of fatigue—a state in which the individual feels only half alive. There are three major types of fatigue: neuromuscular, which is related to poor endurance in muscular performance; organic, which is related to the autonomic, or involuntary, nervous system and the viscera; and finally, mental fatigue, which often manifests itself as boredom and which leads to a lowering of morale.

MIDDLE-AGE AILMENTS.   More serious than fatigue are the ailments which commonly attack the middle-aged body. The list is long and unpleasant. It includes poor posture, painful feet, diges-

tive disorders, headaches, neurasthenia, insomnia, fatty degener-
ation of muscles, a soft protruding abdominal wall, breathlessness
from slight exertion, sex disfunction, piles, ulcers, undernourish-
ment and severe muscular soreness after moderate exercise.

If you recognize any of these ailments as being your own, you
can consider it a possible sign of your poor physical condition.
It is particularly important to be alert to these symptoms because
they are not only undesirable in themselves, they are also the
forerunners of more serious ailments, like prostate disease, kidney
disease, heart disease, cancer and many others.

As you can see, the consequences of physical decline can be
dramatic and serious. But rather than frighten you with dire fore-
bodings, it will be far more helpful and constructive if you can
understand how and why your body ages and degenerates.

THE ROLE OF THE BLOODSTREAM.   Although many things make for
a well-conditioned body, perhaps the key is the circulatory system. No part of the human body can thrive, or even survive,
without the service of the heart and the bloodstream.

Why this is so is obvious when you consider the job that the
bloodstream performs. It carries nutriment and oxygen to every
cell of the body and exchanges them for waste materials, which it
helps dispose of. It distributes hormones throughout the body so
that many important functions can be performed. And, with the
aid of its white blood corpuscles, the bloodstream fights infectious
diseases.

CIRCULATORY DECLINE.   Under adverse conditions the circulatory
system deteriorates in two principal ways: From thickening or
hardening of the walls of the blood vessels it can decline in its
ability to transport blood efficiently; and it can shrink in total
volume when blood is not permitted to flow freely through certain
areas of the body—by inactivity, poor posture, unnatural pres-
sures and so on.

It is easy to imagine the theoretical results of circulatory deterioration. Without access to the bloodstream, a living cell is cut
off from its supply of nutriment and oxygen. It can then no longer
live. Without an efficient bloodstream the body cannot fight disease effectively. Regulation of vital physical functions by hormones can no longer occur efficiently.

By no means everything is understood about the biochemistry of physical decline and the onset of disease, but it is evident from observation that decline of the circulatory system is accompanied by *loss of endurance,* less resistance to *fatigue,* more susceptibility to *stress* and greater vulnerability to *disease.*

THE ADVANTAGES OF GOOD CIRCULATION.   These conclusions are supported by the performances under stress of people who have maintained sound circulatory fitness through active lives. At the Fitness Center we have frequently noted while testing people in varying degrees of fitness that those who showed more relaxed blood vessels, less circulatory ptosis (imbalance of blood distribution in the body) and superior blood flow scored significantly higher in tests of strength and endurance. This was reflected in all tests, but especially, and perhaps most dramatically, after hard treadmill running, cycling and rowing.

GREATER ENDURANCE.   There are countless other indications that people engaged in activities that require maximum performance of the circulatory system are better able to withstand fatigue, disease and physical hardship. Consider, for example, the company of 2,200 men serving under a Colonel William R. Rutherford in the Cherokee Indian War of 1776, who, according to a history of South Carolina, marched over the Great Smoky Mountains and lived in the wilderness for a year without anything resembling the shelter known to modern soldiers. They ate whatever they could wrest from the wilderness; they lived in the snow for many months. Yet not one single man died from disease of any kind.

This seems a remarkable record, especially to the modern observer. One can only conclude that the daily program of marching, foraging, working, hauling equipment and fighting kept the men in peak physical condition and served as a form of preventive medicine.

RESISTANCE TO DISEASE.   We can even speculate that maintenance of sound circulatory condition forestalls the onset of serious chronic diseases. We have no proof or real understanding of this yet, but health educators and departments of social medicine are studying this theory.

Only time and human research will establish the validity of such speculation. In the meantime we will have to be satisfied with our modest observations. These include the obvious connections between good circulation and heart disease, stomach and duodenal ulcers and the painful effects of swelling tissues.

THE CAUSES OF CIRCULATORY DECLINE.   Having now made a strong case for the benefits of maintaining a fit circulatory system, it remains for us to learn how to go about achieving such fitness. To do so, we should first have some idea of what causes circulatory deterioration.

The general cause of decline is what in medicine is called stress, which is simply a convenient way to describe the general wear and tear of living. Obviously, some stress cannot be avoided in the process of living. That is why the human body ages, no matter how well it is cared for. But the degree of stress to which the body is subjected can be varied and controlled.

STRESS.   The greatest stress takes the form of unnatural treatment of the body. Unnatural treatment includes such things as overeating, staying in a cramped position for long intervals, extended overexcitement and, more obviously, introducing large quantities of toxic substances like alcohol or nicotine into the system.

Daily life in contemporary America involves unnatural stress. Living under the pressure of a crowded schedule of appointments, deadlines and other responsibilities is likely to create a state of anxiety which will cause "vasoconstriction" (tense blood vessels), high blood pressure, and consequently, a less efficient bloodstream. Increased anxiety frequently leads to overconsumption of food, alcohol and nicotine. Overeating causes the body to store away as fatty tissue food that it can't burn in activity, which in turn puts an added burden on the circulatory system by forcing it to supply nourishment to a larger area. Alcohol and nicotine cut down the system's efficiency. Fatigue sets in; anxiety increases; we are caught in a vicious cycle which can only lead to a massive physical breakdown.

Graphic illustration of this process can be seen daily in newspaper obituaries reporting deaths from heart attack of people in their late thirties and early forties. The earlier stages of the process are reflected in tests like the ones performed by Dr. Hardin Jones of the University of California. After examining 500 workers, Dr. Jones found that the average eighteen year old has 25 cubic centimeters of blood passing through each single liter of muscle tissue. At the age of twenty-five, this figure drops to 16 cc. per liter, or a decline of roughly 40 per cent. And by thirty-five, it's down to 10 cc.—60 per cent less!

Clearly, when it comes to physical fitness there is more to worry about than one's appearance. But the logic of what we have seen also points to the conclusion that if a half-alive state of existence and ill health are the results of physical decline, then both can be avoided by maintaining physical fitness.

The truth of this logic is demonstrated in the next chapter.

3. The Benefits of Exercise

WORK CAN MAKE YOU YOUNGER.   If you will summon up that clichéd picture of the feeble old man, aged before his time by endless hours of manual labor, you will be surprised when we state that hard work is the secret to staying young. Nevertheless, it's true that with the proper program of real physical exertion a person can not only avoid feebleness, he can actually reverse the aging process and regain a certain amount of his youth.

At the Physical Fitness Center some years ago, we examined a large number of former athletic champions who had reached middle age. Some members of this group had kept up reasonably regular physical training, while others had given up exercising completely. We compared the results of the examinations with those of examinations of a group of younger athletes. Among the older group, those who had kept in shape were almost on a physical par with the younger group; those who had given up training showed marked deterioration and loss of function, and were dramatically different from the younger group.

On paper the foregoing illustration looks obvious and cut and dried. I only wish the reader could have seen the difference in appearance between the two groups of older men.

To give one further illustration, let's consider two other cases from our files. Many years ago there were two swimmers of great ability. For a period of some years they had been among the best competitors around; each won many races and almost matched the other in ability. One of them eventually gave up swimming and went into business. He was successful, but took no exercise except a little casual golf and he indulged in moderate social drinking. In a period of a dozen years he gained 75 pounds. He died at the age of forty-two.

The other man continued to swim as much as possible, adopted a year-round program of exercise, and at the same time became a successful business executive. Today he is in his seventies and in fine condition, having put on very little weight, and is still able to swim the crawl stroke for 1500 meters.

The conclusion is inescapable and needs little elaboration: When it comes to physical fitness and health, to let nature take its course is to travel a shortcut to the grave. But rather than trundle out any more hobgoblins to frighten you, let's have a closer look at the physiology of fitness and what effects vigorous exercise have on the human body.

EXERCISE AND THE CIRCULATORY SYSTEM.   First of all, let's consider the effect of exercise on that most essential part of the human body, the circulatory system. We have already described how much physical condition depends on the soundness of the circulation. If it can be demonstrated that exercise has a beneficial effect on the function of the circulatory system, then one of the routes to improved health will become clear.

Contrary to popular notion, the heart is a muscle that (like all muscles) improves with work. Its ability to pump blood through arteries and veins—keeping them flexible—depends not so much on how old you are as it does on what chance you give your heart to work. The small blood vessels must also be kept open, and the best way to do this is to make the heart work harder.

The regenerative capacity of the circulatory system can be illustrated by the fact that, frequently, a person who has gone through thirty or forty minutes of warm-up exercises will have lower blood pressure than he had before he started exercising.

This drop in blood pressure results from blood being forced into capillaries which were previously closed. By opening up and dilating inactive capillaries the total volume of the bloodstream is increased. The result is lower blood pressure.

PRACTICAL BENEFITS.   One practical result of this expansion of the bloodstream is that parts of the body which had not previously been directly supplied with blood gain direct access to the body's vital fluid. New cells, and therefore new tissue, can then develop.

An improved circulatory system also means that the body can carry out other functions more efficiently. The whole metabolism improves; the body develops greater resistance to stress; the aging process is slowed down.

Improved circulation means that oxygen can be transported from the alveoli of the lungs to remote parts of the body more rapidly. Since muscular fatigue results from a diminished supply of oxygen, it is obvious that better circulation means greater strength, more endurance and improved motor fitness.

All of the foregoing explains why a person who exercises regularly and vigorously will find himself getting steadily stronger and more fit.

Another way that a person reaps the harvest of vigorous exercise is in reduced tension and fatigue. As the Mayo Clinic announced some years ago, chronic fatigue is seldom relieved by rest and sleep. Some 5 to 10 per cent of all adults who came to the Mayo Clinic were suffering from the chronic type of fatigue that produces a tired, anxious, fretful state of mind that in turn prevents the individual from being able to sleep, eat, or work with satisfaction, and who is increasingly sensitive, tense and introverted. It was found that buoyant energetic health—the very opposite of fatigue—resulted from a program of physical exertion.

The cumulative effect of these various benefits of exercise is very often a marked improvement in a person's mental state. While it is increasingly apparent that one's emotional state can govern one's physical condition, the opposite is also true in some cases. Proper exercise affects the endocrine glands, and the glands are closely tied up with the emotions.

To state our case in the most dramatic terms: Exercise can make you feel like a new person. Very likely you will become more alert and have a sense of being more alive. Everything you experience will take on new meaning; you'll be less irritable and "jumpy"; you'll be able to work harder and play with greater enjoyment; you'll enjoy life more.

EXERCISE AND ILLNESS.   It is even possible that a planned program of physical activity helps people recovering from some forms of disease. In the past it has been the tendency of practicing physicians who work closely with sick patients to minimize the importance of exercise. Recently, however, exercise has been increasingly recommended for patients convalescing from such diseases as rheumatic fever, heart disease and various types of injuries. More and more, special convalescing exercises are begun while the patient is still in bed, and increased very slowly as the patient regains his strength.

Doctors who have studied the value of exercise are now regularly prescribing it for low backache, insomnia, chronic headache, low metabolism, nervous anxiety and dozens of kindred disorders which do not seem to have a direct germinal or virus cause.

In my own experience, I would cite the case of a young man in Finland—a former athlete—who told me that a few years after he had given up his athletic career he suffered from the onset of rather severe arthritis. Speculating that his affliction might have something to do with the sedentary nature of his new occupation, he began a program of daily running. After a few months he found his arthritis greatly reduced.

He has continued his routine of moderate running for ten years now, and he has found his arthritis virtually eliminated.

At the Center, in addition to measuring gains in physical fitness, we make a point of asking people if they have noticed any effects that exercise has had upon chronic ailments. We have had remarkable testimony to the value of exercise in reducing a variety of afflictions, including colds, backaches, insomnia, chronic fatigue, nervous tension, sexual impotence and a host of chronic problems which can usually be traced to poor circulation.

Over the years I have grown more and more impressed by the widespread positive results of vigorous˙exercise. I will not be at all surprised to learn of scientific substantiation of our observations in the near future.

4. What About You?

APPEARANCES DON'T REVEAL MUCH.   Now that you have a more detailed idea of what it means to be physically fit, take the first opportunity you have to strip down and look at yourself in a full-length mirror.

Actually, what you see won't tell you very much. Your external appearance just doesn't reflect the true state of your bloodstream, and it is this, not the firmness of your muscles or the excellence of your physique, which determines your true degree of fitness.

EXTREME SYMPTOMS.   Nevertheless, there are some extreme external conditions which you should look out for. An excessively soft and protruding abdomen usually indicates poor circulation and a pooling of blood in the internal organs, accompanied by exceedingly poor organic endurance.

If you take measurements of your chest fully expanded, and your stomach in a normal position, and find that your abdominal girth is larger than the girth of your chest, it is a bad sign. In fact, statistically, your chances of dying prematurely are two-and-a-quarter times those of the man of average proportions.

If your weight is one-third or more greater than the average for a person of your height and morphological type, you fall into a category where the death rate is one-and-a-half times that of the average.

But aside from these extreme symptoms, there isn't a great deal that you can tell about your physical condition from your appearance.

MORPHOLOGICAL TYPES.   Every individual adheres to his own morphological type, which he can no more change than the color of his skin or the size of his bones. That is why there are some people who will never run a mile in under four minutes or play center for the Boston Celtics.

MUSCULARITY.   Even an impressive physique, like the ones that adorn the covers of muscle magazines, are not an indication of good physical condition. Muscular "definition," as it is sometimes referred to, does not reflect true muscular strength. Furthermore, even muscular strength is not a true indication of useful physical fitness. Muscular strength alone does not enable a person to resist fatigue or disease.

As we have shown, physical fitness depends essentially on the condition of the circulatory system—the ability of the bloodstream to pick up oxygen from the alveoli of the lungs and to transfer it to the working cells of the muscles.

PHYSICAL FITNESS TESTS.   At the Physical Fitness Center, we have one hundred and twenty-eight tests that measure every aspect of physical fitness. To pass these tests requires agility, endurance, strength, balance, flexibility and power. By putting a person through these tests, we can draw an exhaustively detailed profile of his physical condition.

From these tests we have derived a series of simpler tests which you take in your own home, so that you can get an idea of your own comparative condition. These tests are presented in the next section of this book.

Section II

HOW TO TEST

YOUR PHYSICAL

CONDITION

5. What Physical Fitness Is

This section contains two series of tests. Both are designed so that you can take them in your own home. One will help you to determine your general physical condition; the other is a simplified test of what we refer to as your motor fitness. As you will see, the test of motor fitness is actually a detailed examination of various aspects of your physical fitness. Before we come to the test of motor fitness, we shall examine in more detail what motor fitness means.

As for physical fitness: By now you will understand that your physical fitness can be described in so many different ways—the condition of your circulatory system, your resistance to fatigue, your ability to withstand disease, your general state of mind and so on—that the only way to define it is in pretty general terms.

Over the years, I have come to look upon physical fitness as the trunk of a tree that supports the many branches which represent all the activities that make life worth living: intellectual life, spiritual life, occupation, love life and social activities.

Let something happen to the trunk of the tree that weakens it and all the rest of the tree will wither and finally perish.

To say this in more straightforward language, and to recapitulate what has already been said, being in good physical condition enables a person to withstand stress, thus making him resistant to fatigue and the many mild infections which afflict the fatigued person. Similarly, a person whose body has not been weakened by minor infections will have more energy to cope with life.

Physical fitness—along with the desire for health that should be part of it—also enables a person to avoid psychosomatic ailments. It makes it possible for the mind and the body to work together as if integrated by a drive shaft. The normal aging process corrodes this drive shaft, so that the body no longer obeys the mind. Proper physical training has the effect of lubricating the drive shaft.

Obviously, there is no precise and completely reliable way of gauging a person's physical fitness. The real test is intuitive, and the truly fit person can know that he is truly fit only by sensing that he is deriving the most possible satisfaction from living.

I do not mean to suggest that the physically fit person should be happy all the time. Nobody who is experiencing life completely can be happy all the time. I only mean that his senses should be alive, his feelings complete, and his awareness of the world around him as finely tuned as possible.

6. Ten Simple Ways to Test Your Physical Fitness

As we mentioned earlier, at our Center we have as many as one hundred and twenty-eight tests to measure every area of physical fitness. The following ten tests, which are selected and adapted from our larger group of tests, are designed to enable you to get an idea of your own condition.

Each of the tests is worth a certain number of points, if you are able to pass it. Take the entire battery of tests, and write your scores down as you go along. When you have finished, add up your scores to get your total. A perfect score is 200 points. The average is around 100 points. Any score below 100 can be considered a failure and is an indication of poor physical condition.

STANDARD TEST OF GENERAL PHYSICAL FITNESS

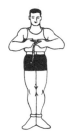

1. SCORE: 25 POINTS   **YOUR SCORE: ___**

Stand with your shoulders back and your chest expanded to the maximum degree. Measure the circumference of your chest just beneath your armpits. Then measure your waist, with your stomach in a relaxed position—not sucked in or forced out. Your chest should measure 5 inches more than your waist. (For women, the difference should be 10 inches.)

2. SCORE: 10 POINTS   **YOUR SCORE: ___**

Sit on the floor with your legs stretched out in front of you, and place an 8-inch-high book upright between your knees. Then, keeping your legs straight and flat on the floor, bend forward and touch your forehead to the top of the book.

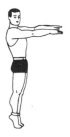

3. SCORE: 15 POINTS   **YOUR SCORE: ___**

Stand on your toes, with your heels together, your eyes closed, and your arms extended forward at the shoulders. Stay in this position for 20 seconds without shifting your feet or opening your eyes.

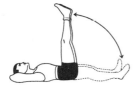

4. SCORE: 20 POINTS   YOUR SCORE: ___

Lie on your back with your hands behind your neck, and raise both legs to a vertical position without bending them at the knees. Then lower your legs to the floor, again without bending them at the knees. Repeat this 20 times successively.

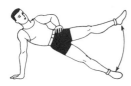

5. SCORE: 15 POINTS   YOUR SCORE: ___

Support your body stretched straight and sideways on one hand (with your arm held straight) and the outside of one foot. Place your other hand on your hip. Raise your upper leg to a horizontal position 25 times, without bending either knee.

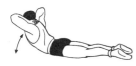

6. SCORE: 25 POINTS   YOUR SCORE: ___

Lying flat on your stomach, face down, with your fingers laced behind your neck and your feet pinned to the floor, raise your chin until it is 18 inches off the floor.

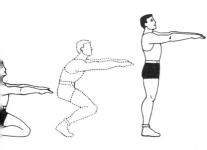

7. SCORE: 10 POINTS   YOUR SCORE: ___

From a kneeling position, with the soles of your feet up and your arms stretched forward from the shoulders, swing arms down and up, jump to a standing position, and hold your balance. Both feet should come up together.

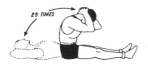

8. SCORE: 20 POINTS   YOUR SCORE: ___

Lie on your back with your hands behind your neck, your legs straight, and free (not held down). Do 25 sit-ups without pausing for rest.

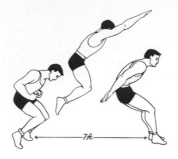

9. SCORE: 10 POINTS   YOUR SCORE: ___

Do a standing broad jump. Do *not* take a running start. The length of your jump should approximately equal your height.

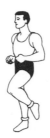

10. SCORE: 50 POINTS   YOUR SCORE: ___

Run in place for 60 seconds, lifting your feet at least 4 inches from the floor. Then take 3 deep breaths. Then hold your breath for 60 seconds.

YOUR TOTAL SCORE: ___

How many of the above tests did you pass? What was your total score? A perfect score, as we said, is 200 points. The average is 100 points.

If your total is below 100, you are in poor shape and urgently in need of an intensive conditioning program. If you failed the last test, and any other two, you should seriously consider a physical conditioning program. Even if you did fairly well, a good conditioning program will enable you to hold on to your present condition, and even improve it.

We will outline several training programs later in this book. Before we proceed, however, we shall present a more extensive series of eighteen tests which you can take to get a more detailed picture of your physical condition. These tests are designed to measure your balance, flexibility, agility, strength, power and endurance—or what we call your motor fitness.

7. *What Motor Fitness Is*

When we speak of *motor fitness,* we are referring to the specific physical aspects of fitness—the ability to perform certain actions, including the capacity to run, jump, dodge, fall, climb, swim, ride, lift and carry heavy loads, and endure long hours of continuous work. Motor fitness has to do with the physical abilities which are dominated by the kinesthetic sense—that is, the muscle sense—the body's muscular energy and the suppleness of the tissues and joints. Any test of motor fitness involves the big muscles of the body which are used in athletic or work skills, rather than those used in finer, low-energy, precision skills.

Motor fitness includes balance, flexibility, agility, strength, power and endurance.

BALANCE.   The ability to balance is the result of neuromuscular control—that is, the nerves and muscles working collectively when we perform actions like skating, riding, skiing, dancing and many everyday skills.

Many people find themselves handicapped by a tendency to fall and get hurt at the slightest provocation. They cannot step on a rug without slipping; they injure themselves in the shower, or when they get out of a moving vehicle.

We refer to a person with this tendency as being "accident prone," and let it go at that. But accident proneness results from poor awareness of bodily movements, from unsteadiness and from lack of control. At bottom is simply a lack of balance.

A faulty sense of balance can be remedied. Improved sense of the body—or kinesthetic sense—can be developed by a variety of balancing exercises. These will be found in the fundamental gymnastic program described later in this book.

FLEXIBILITY.   Flexibility has to do with a person's ability to move his joints. A flexible body is able to perform a wide range of movements—to tuck up tightly, to bend easily at the waist, to twist the spine, to point the toes inward and outward and to breathe deeply with little extra effort. Flexibility indicates that the joints are not muscle-bound or stiff for some other reason.

It takes physical flexibility to jump a hurdle, to crawl through a culvert, to jump over a stick held in the hands, to skin the cat or do fancy diving. Obviously, the average person doesn't have to perform such feats very often. Only soldiers and athletes require this kind of flexibility. But you need a certain amount of flexibility to walk smoothly, to sit down or stand up with grace, to stand in a moving subway or bus. And people with poor flexibility usually tire easily and are more prone to illness and accidents.

AGILITY.   Agility may be described as the ability to react quickly with controlled and nimble movements. It takes agility to dodge a ball, to spring quickly to one's feet, to climb up a cargo net swiftly, to run and weave through a maze of obstacles, to vault fences or barriers, to lie down and get up quickly, or to jump onto a horse or a vehicle.

Not exactly activities you're likely to be doing today or tomorrow. Nevertheless, these are some of the things which we require people to do at the Center. The idea is to develop the abilities that are required in emergencies—to climb out of a burning plane, to pull oneself into a lifeboat, to climb a rope onto a ship, or to lower oneself by rope from a burning building.

A person who can control his body quickly and efficiently has the power to save both himself and others in an emergency. More important, agility gives a person the chance to do more without running the risk of getting hurt.

STRENGTH.   Strength refers to the ability of the hands, legs or trunk to exert force.

Strong hands and arms are important for grasping, lifting or pulling heavy or resistant objects. Strong feet and legs are needed to bear the weight of the body, in addition to carrying extra burdens. Weak feet and legs are a handicap to walking or marching, even without a load. Obviously, strong legs and feet are required for such activities as jumping, running, skating or skiing.

Most important of all is strength of the trunk. The trunk is the base from which the arm and thigh muscles arise, and therefore must support any exertions of the arms and legs. The muscles of the upper part of the back and the chest are essential to chinning or climbing. The muscles of the buttocks play a role in most forms of locomotion, including running, jumping and cycling. The long back muscles hold the trunk erect and help to steady it while the body pushes or pulls. The abdominal and thigh flexor muscles reinforce all kicking movements, and aid the body in performing sit-ups and leg-lifting movements.

A person who lacks strength may be severely handicapped. In extreme cases he may be unable to sit up from a prone position or lift his legs from the floor while lying on his back. He will find it difficult to perform hundreds of everyday tasks which he normally takes for granted as being easy to do.

POWER.   Power is the aspect of motor fitness which describes the capacity to release a great amount of force with a sudden exertion. Power is a key ingredient in successfully performing sports. It takes power to high jump, sprint, pole vault or broad jump. Many phases of football and baseball require power. Power can be thought of as that element which thrusts the entire body forward suddenly, or which is needed to propel some object independent of the body, like a ball or a javelin.

ENDURANCE.   Last and perhaps most important is endurance—the capacity for continued exertion in spite of a severe depletion of the oxygen reserve of the body during the first minute or two of activity. A person is able to overcome this initial phase of fatigue through deep breathing and the capacity of the circulatory system to speed up its job of supplying oxygen to the working muscle cells. The feeling of relief that results when the body has adapted itself is commonly referred to as "second wind."

The most obvious tests of endurance are long-distance running, swimming, mountain climbing and marching long distances with a heavy load.

Balance, flexibility, agility, strength, power and endurance: These are the six cardinal points in our system of motor fitness. These are the things that the next simplified series of tests will rate you on.

8. Eighteen Simple Ways to Test Your Motor Fitness

Each of the following eighteen tests is designed to test one of the six aspects of motor fitness, as you will see. Unlike the previous tests, each test counts one point. You will figure your score on the basis of how many out of the eighteen tests you passed.

THREE BALANCE TESTS:

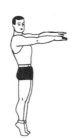

1. Stand on your toes, with your heels together, your eyes closed, and your arms stretched forward at the shoulders. Stay in this position for 20 seconds without shifting your feet or opening your eyes. (This test is the same as Test 3 of the first series.)

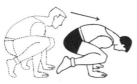

2. Assume a squatting position, with your palms flat on the floor and your arms between your bent legs so that your elbows are touching your legs just below your knees. Now tip forward, put the full weight of your body on your arms and hands, and lift yourself so that your toes are off the floor and your body is balanced on your hands. (As you tip forward, you will find it necessary to rest your legs on your elbows.) Hold this balancing position for 20 seconds.

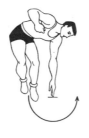

3. Bend down and touch the floor with one index finger. Then walk in a circle around your finger 10 times. (Imagine that your finger is one leg of a compass and the rest of your body is the other leg, and that you are drawing a circle around the central point represented by your finger.) After you have completed 10 turns, preferably within 30 seconds, walk a straight 10-foot line within 5 seconds, keeping each foot squarely on the line.

THREE FLEXIBILITY TESTS:

4. Keeping your legs together and your knees locked, bend at the waist and touch the floor with your fingertips. (Women should touch the floor with their palms.)

5. Sit on the floor with your legs stretched out in front of you, and place an 8-inch-high book upright between your knees. Then, keeping your legs straight and flat on the floor, bend forward and touch your forehead to the top of the book. (This test is the same as Test 2 of the first series.)

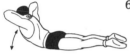

6. Lying flat on your stomach, face down, with your fingers laced behind your neck and your feet pinned to the floor, raise your chin until it is 18 inches off the floor. (This test is the same as Test 6 of the first series.)

THREE AGILITY TESTS:

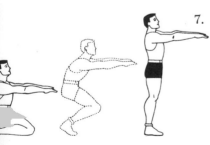

7. From a kneeling position, with the soles of your feet up and your arms stretched forward from the shoulders, swing arms up, jump to a standing position, and hold your balance. Both feet should come up together. (This test is the same as Test 7 of the first series.)

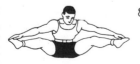

8. From a standing position, leap off the floor and touch your toes with your fingertips, without bending your legs. Repeat 5 times in 5 seconds.

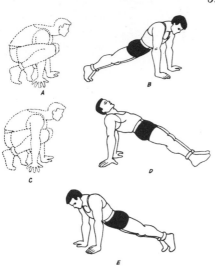

9. Assume a squatting position, with your palms flat against the floor, your arms straight, and your knees outside your elbows. Next, with the weight of your body resting on your hands, kick backward so that your legs are extended full length. Next, return to a squatting position, with your knees *between* your elbows, and then kick forward so that your legs are extended full length in front of you and you are resting on your back, with your weight on your hands and heels. Then, shifting your weight to one arm, turn yourself over so that you are facing the ground once more, return to your original squatting position, and stand up. Repeat this procedure 6 times in 20 seconds. (Women taking this exercise should simply squat, extend legs backward, return to squat, and stand—6 times in 10 seconds.)

THREE STRENGTH TESTS:

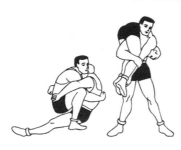

10. If convenient, select a partner who weighs within 10 pounds of what you weigh, lift him, and balance him across your shoulders. You should perform the lift within 10 seconds.

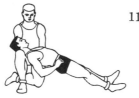

11. In the back leaning rest position, with your heels on the floor, your head on your partner's knee (or the edge of a chair or sofa) and your hands on your hips, hold your body rigid for 30 seconds.

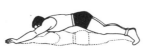

12. Lie face downward. With your arms extended forward full length, your elbows and knees rigid, lift your body by pressing down on your palms, until you are balanced on your hands and your toes. Raise your abdomen 4 inches from the floor. (Women should use forearms instead of palms, and hold position for 20 seconds.)

A POWER TEST:

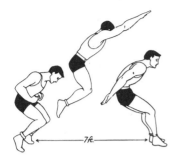

13. Do a standing broad jump. Do *not* take a running start. The length of your jump should approximately equal your height. (If you are under twenty-five years old, add one foot.) (This test is the same as Test 9 of the first series.)

FIVE ENDURANCE TESTS:

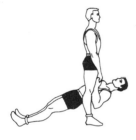

14. Do 15 full-length push-ups, starting from a prone position, with the hands positioned beneath shoulders. (Women should do 30, keeping knees on the floor.)

15. Lie on your back, straddled by a standing partner. Grasp his hands with your own hands and pull yourself up until your chest strikes his legs (the higher the better). Repeat 20 times. (Women should repeat 10 times.)

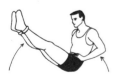

16. Sit on the floor, with your trunk straight upright, your legs outstretched, your knees stiff, and your hands on your hips. Then lean back so that your legs come off the floor. With your knees remaining rigid, hold this V-position for 60 seconds.

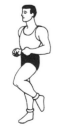

17. Run in place for 2 minutes, doing 180 steps per minute. Then hold your breath for 30 seconds.

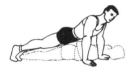

18. In succession, do 200 two-footed hops, 200 straddle jumps (jumping alternately with feet together and apart), 200 alternate stride hops (reversing feet scissor-style on each hop), and 50 hops on each foot.

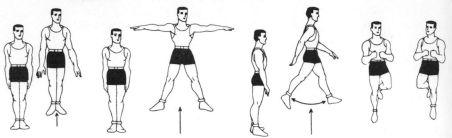

Unless you are in good shape, and accustomed to exercising vigorously every day, the chances are you will not have passed more than 10 of these 18 exercises.

The average adult male over twenty-five years old will pass only 9 of the 18 tests. If you can do 10 out of the 18, you are above average.

To help you judge your own performance more accurately, here is how the majority of normal young adults performed in this series of tests at the University of Illinois' Physical Fitness Research Center:

The men generally passed Tests 1, 4, 5, 7, 10, 11, 13, 14, 15 and 16. They failed Tests 2, 3, 6, 8, 9, 12, 17 and 18.

The women generally passed Tests 1, 3, 4, 5, 7, 8, 9, 10, 12 and 14. They failed Tests 2, 6, 11, 13, 15, 16, 17 and 18.

In most cases the variation between men's and women's performances can be explained by the difference in basic physical attributes. In all cases, however, the failure to pass a certain test is an indication of some lack of motor fitness.

9. How to Test Your Cardiovascular Fitness

Before we enter into the more practical phase of this book, we are going to describe a number of tests that you can take to evaluate your cardiovascular fitness.

Cardiovascular fitness simply describes the capacity, endurance and efficiency of your circulatory system—or the ability of your bloodstream to transport oxygen from the alveoli of your lungs to the muscle cells of your body.

Two of the following tests—the Breath-Holding Test and the Progressive Pulse-Ratio Test—are useful gauges for evaluating the condition of your cardiovascular system, regardless of whether or not you are "in shape." The other tests described in this chapter are more specialized; they should only be taken after a period of training, preferably under professional supervision.

THE BREATH–HOLDING TEST

One simple and acceptable way of testing your respiratory capacity, which is related to circulatory fitness, is to step onto and off of a chair, bench or stool (approximately 17 inches high for men; 14 inches high for women) for a period of one minute, and then to see how long you can hold your breath. You should be able to hold it for at least thirty seconds. If you can't, it's an indication that your cardiovascular condition has deteriorated below a desirable level.

THE PROGRESSIVE PULSE–RATIO TEST

The progressive pulse-ratio test is a simple but extremely valuable method of measuring your capacity to utilize oxygen during physical exertion. It is a middle-gear test, designed for people who are not in top physical condition. Ideally, the test should be administered by trained personnel, but it can be taken with the assistance of a friend, providing the instructions are followed carefully.

1. Begin by sitting relaxed for five minutes. Then take your pulse rate, in the sitting position, for fifteen seconds. Note on a piece of paper the number of pulse beats you counted. After a thirty-second interval, take your pulse rate again for fifteen seconds. If the two readings are the same, your pulse is stable and you can proceed with the test. If the readings are different, you should continue taking readings at thirty-second intervals until two successive counts are the same. If slight fluctuations continue, an average figure should be noted.

2. Stand up, and step onto and off of a chair, bench or stool (approximately 17 inches high for men; 14 inches high for women) 12 times in one minute. (Each "round trip" should take five seconds. Have someone time you and call off five-second intervals, so that you can pace yourself. Count to yourself the number of "trips" you make.) When you have completed 12 "trips" on and off the chair, sit down, wait ten seconds, then take another pulse reading, for a two-minute period, and note *directly above* the first reading the number of pulse beats that occurred during the period. (You should now have a notation approximately like the following, except that the amounts will be different: $\frac{123}{56}$)

3. After a five-minute rest interval, recheck your resting pulse rate for a fifteen-second period at thirty-second intervals until you get two readings alike and the rate is stable again. Record this reading to the right of your original resting pulse reading. (i.e. $\frac{123}{56}\ \frac{}{56}$)

4. Stand up again, and step onto and off of the chair 18 times in one minute. (This time, each "trip" should take about three-and-a-third seconds.) Sit down, take your pulse for another two minutes, and record this reading directly over your second resting-pulse reading.

5. After a five-minute interval, recheck your resting pulse rate for a fifteen-second period at thirty-second intervals until you get two readings alike and the rate is stable again: Record this reading to the right of your second resting pulse reading.

6. Step onto and off of the chair 24 times in one minute (at the rate of two-and-a-half seconds per "trip"). Sit down, take your pulse for another two minutes, and record this reading directly over your third resting-pulse reading.

7. After a five-minute interval, recheck your resting pulse rate (as in step 5) until it is stable again. Record this reading to the right of your third resting pulse reading.

8. Step onto and off of the chair 30 times in one minute (at the rate of two seconds per "trip"). Sit down, take your pulse rate for another two minutes, and record this reading directly over your fourth resting pulse reading.

9. After a five-minute interval, recheck your sitting pulse rate

until it is stable again (as in step 7). Record this reading to the right of your fourth resting pulse reading.

10. Step onto and off of the chair 36 times in one minute (at the rate of three "trips" every five seconds). Sit down, take your pulse rate for another two minutes, and record this reading directly over your fifth resting pulse reading.

You should now have a list of figures that might look approximately like the following, depending on what kind of condition you are in:

2 Minute Count	123	135	141	163	241
Resting Pulse (15 secs.)	56	56	56	60	64

Now divide each lower number (the resting-pulse) into the number above it (the two-minute count). The results will be a series of ratios. In this hypothetical case, the figures would read as follows:

Ratio	2.20	2.41	2.52	2.72	3.77

If you wish to get a clearer picture of the results of your test, you can sketch a simple graph, letting the vertical axis represent Pulse Ratios (from 2.00 to 4.00), and letting the horizon axis represent Steps Per Minute (from 12 to 36). (Printed forms of such a graph are available at many Y.M.C.A.'s throughout the country.) Plot your five pulse-ratio figures on the graph and connect the five points with lines.

EVALUATING THE RESULTS.   A person with a high degree of cardiovascular fitness will have little trouble taking in oxygen under increasingly strenuous conditions. As he increases the rate of his activity, his circulatory system is able to supply more oxygen without noticeably speeding up its activity. His pulse rate, which is the measure of the bloodstream's activity, remains the same. When he rests, his pulse rate quickly returns to its normal resting pace.

You can see that a physically fit person who takes the Progressive Pulse-Ratio Test and feels little strain as the pace quickens will have fairly constant pulse readings. And because the increasing pace will have little effect on him, his two-minute count after exertion will change very little. As a result, his pulse ratio will vary only slightly. And the line on his graph will rise very gradually. As a matter of fact, the graphic lines of championship athletes that we have tested are invariably straight and almost horizontal.

On the other hand, when a person in poor physical condition increases the rate of his exertion, his system must work harder and harder to get the necessary oxygen. The rate of his pulse increases sharply; his pulse ratio gets greater; and his "line" on the graph will rise steeply. If he reaches the limit of his oxygen intake capacity, begins to get fatigued, and grows tense, the plotted pulse-ratio line will "break," that is, turn sharply upward in a deviation from the slope determined by the first two or three points.

You can evaluate your own results by comparing them with the figures on the charts below, which were prepared from the results of testing hundreds of men and women over a period of several years.

ADULT MEN (26–60 years old)

Classification	Ratio for 12 steps per min.	Ratio for 18 steps per min.	Ratio for 24 steps per min.	Ratio for 30 steps per min.	Ratio for 36 steps per min.	Percentile
Excellent	1.72 to 1.80	1.73 to 1.84	1.72 to 1.88	1.79 to 1.98	1.62 to 1.90	99.9 to 99.2
Above Average	1.85 to 2.07	1.90 to 2.19	1.95 to 2.34	2.07 to 2.54	2.03 to 2.73	98 to 72
Average	2.11 to 2.20	2.24 to 2.36	2.42 to 2.57	2.63 to 2.82	2.87 to 3.15	61 to 38
Below Average	2.24 to 2.46	2.42 to 2.70	2.65 to 3.03	2.92 to 3.39	3.28 to 3.98	27 to 1.8
Poor	2.50 to 2.59	2.76 to 2.88	3.11 to 3.26	3.48 to 3.67	4.12 to 4.40	.82 to .14

ADULT WOMEN (26–60 years old)

Classification	Ratio for 12 steps per min.	Ratio for 18 steps per min.	Ratio for 24 steps per min.	Ratio for 30 steps per min.	Ratio for 36 steps per min.	Percentile
Excellent	1.59 to 1.71	1.63 to 1.77	1.76 to 1.92	1.79 to 1.99	1.95 to 2.16	99.9 to 99.2
Above Average	1.77 to 2.06	1.84 to 2.19	2.00 to 2.39	2.10 to 2.61	2.26 to 2.77	98.2 to 72.6
Average	2.12 to 2.23	2.26 to 2.40	2.47 to 2.63	2.71 to 2.92	2.87 to 3.07	61.8 to 38.2
Below Average	2.29 to 2.58	2.47 to 2.82	2.71 to 3.11	3.02 to 3.53	3.17 to 3.68	27.4 to 1.8
Poor	2.64 to 2.75	2.89 to 3.03	3.19 to 3.35	3.63 to 3.84	3.78 to 3.99	0.8 to 0.1

THE FIVE–MINUTE STEP TEST

Often referred to as the Harvard Step Test because it was developed at Harvard by Drs. Lucien Brouha and Robert Johnson during the period after World War II, the Five-Minute Step Test is designed to be a high-gear test of cardiovascular condition. It should only be taken by people in top condition, and only under the supervision of trained people.

Check your pulse rate (by counting the number of times it beats in thirty seconds); then place a chair or stool (approximately 17 inches high for men; 14 inches high for women) in front of you and try stepping onto it and off of it, at the rate of 30 times a minute, for five minutes.

At first, you will probably find that you can keep this up for only two or three minutes, but you should add one minute to your time for every month of conditioning you undergo.

When you are able to keep stepping on and off the chair for five consecutive minutes, stop, wait exactly one minute, and check your pulse rate again over a thirty-second interval. Repeat these checks twice more, waiting one minute between each check.

Mark down the number of pulse beats for each of the three thirty-second intervals and add them together for your total score. A score of 111 to 124 is excellent; 131 to 163 is above average; 170 to 183 is average; 190 to 223 is below average; and 229 to 242 is poor. This test will also give you a way to check your progress as you continue your training.

THE ALL–OUT STEP TEST

This test is a high-gear test for people who have had several months of preliminary conditioning and are outstandingly fit. It should not be attempted by beginners, and it should never be attempted without a warm-up period. In addition, a physiologist or a doctor should be present, not only as a safety precaution, but also to take blood-pressure and pulse-rate readings before and after.

The test is taken by stepping onto and off of a chair, bench or stool, at the rate of thirty-six to forty "trips" per minute for as long as the individual can manage.

Doctors, physiologists and physical fitness instructors are developing a great variety of new tests which can measure various aspects of cardiovascular efficiency more and more accurately. Many of these tests are still in the laboratory stage. Nevertheless, the simpler tests described in this chapter can be taken by anyone and will give an idea of general cardiovascular condition.

No matter how well you may have scored on the three series of tests described in this section, it will profit you to read on in the next section, for you will not only find the means to recover your physical fitness, you will also find the means for holding on to the fitness you may have now.

Section III

HOW TO GET BACK

INTO SHAPE

BY YOURSELF

10. Popular Misconceptions about Exercise

A TYPICAL CASE HISTORY.   A few years ago, a fifty-nine-year-old department head at the University of Illinois came to my office seeking help.

He explained that the deaths of several of his friends during the previous year had started him thinking. "I've been leading a pretty sedentary life," he said, "and I don't think it's doing me much good. I've noticed that my feet are weak, my circulation seems to be sluggish, I'm not sleeping well, and I'm overweight. What are the chances of your doing something for someone like me, who's so far over the hill?"

We assured him that there was plenty we could do and went to work. The first thing we established was that the professor had not undertaken any exercise to speak of during the previous five years. He was then given a thorough medical check-up by a physician to make certain he was fundamentally fit to participate in a physical fitness program. In addition, he was given seventy-four tests to appraise his physique, organic efficiency and motor fitness.

Based on the data compiled from the various tests, the following program was outlined for the professor:

1. Two miles of walking per day (to and from work), five days a week.
2. Home calisthenics before breakfast and before going to bed.
3. A daily bath—six days cold and one day hot—followed by vigorous towel rubs.
4. Eighteen holes of golf or a long hike once a week.
5. Ultraviolet-ray treatments three times a week.
6. A diet of reduced fried and starchy foods and increased fruits, vegetables and protein food.

The program was continued for six months, with tests repeated monthly. At the end of the period, the tests indicated that the subject had made important gains in the condition of his physique and cardiovascular system.

His over-all weight decreased only one-and-a-half pounds, but there was a great reduction in fat and a corresponding increase in the strength and density of his muscle tissues—a development usually associated with greatly improved over-all function.

Even more important were the gains recorded in the subject's cardiovascular system. His systolic blood pressure dropped from 142 to 128 in a prone position and from 144 to 124 standing up. His diastolic blood pressure while lying down dropped from 110 to 80, and while standing from 126 to 96. His pulse rate while standing dropped from 82 to 66.

As in all such cases, what these changes reflected could not be established definitely. The routine had either reversed the adult physiological tendency to store fats and inorganic salts in the walls of the blood vessels and in other storage space of the body, or it had simply released him from the kind of psychological tension that constricts the blood vessels.

Suffice it to say that both the professor's physical condition and his state of mind had improved noticeably. And with his decreased blood pressure came the added bonus of increased life expectancy—if life insurance statistics are to be believed.

Whether or not your situation is similar to the professor's, whether you are interested in a physical training program in order to regain fitness or to maintain your present condition, the professor's story raises a number of interesting points.

IT'S NEVER TOO LATE TO BEGIN. We have already seen that physiological middle age does not begin in the forties, as many people think, but midway in the twenties. So the right time to begin work on yourself to counteract and slow up the rate of deterioration is not in your mid-forties, but much earlier.

Nevertheless, as the professor's case illustrates, those people who have neglected to begin actively exercising soon enough and find themselves seriously out of shape in their late forties, fifties and sixties need not give up and say, "I'm too old to begin exercising now."

Some of our brightest "stars" at the Fitness Center have been in their fifties, sixties and seventies. Actually, it is never too late to begin, providing the transition from inactivity to activity is made intelligently.

HARD WORK WON'T KILL YOU. Another misconception about exercise is that "the harder you work, the quicker you die." Not only is this false, it is quite the opposite of the truth. Almost all people must exercise regularly or they degenerate.

Nevertheless, the belief persists that strenuous exercise automatically leads to a heart attack, particularly among older people. This is simply not true. Prominent heart specialists have stated that in normal hearts the muscle fibers are never injured by physical strain. This conclusion is supported by many studies, which indicate that the great majority of normal adult hearts show no appreciable enlargement or injury from the most strenuous sports. In cases where there is enlargement, the heart will reduce to normal size with rest and progressive conditioning exercises.

If strenuous physical exertion does not cause heart disease, then it cannot bring about a heart attack in a healthy system, for the term "heart attack" is only a rather vague description of the most critical stages of heart disease.

It is not exercise that kills people, but the diseases which so often develop from lack of exercise. The heart only functions well if demands are made on it. A soft flabby heart will tire more easily than a strong one; it is less efficient and more susceptible to disease.

USE SOME COMMON SENSE.   Of course, sharp bursts of activity are not always wise. A bookworm whose usual form of exercise consists of walking from the college library to the dining room, or a desk worker whose only form of exercise is an occasional walk to the water cooler or the bus stop, should not suddenly play an hour of tennis or handball at the age of forty-five.

There are many bits of common sense which you should practice before undertaking any strenuous exercise, and we shall discuss them shortly, but first there is one other popular misconception about exercise which should be mentioned.

STREAMLINED EXERCISE PROGRAMS.   In recent years, the country has witnessed the appearance of many exercise programs which guarantee instant fitness in return for only a few minutes of one's daily schedule. The popularity of these programs has many causes, including the government's concern with raising the national fitness standards; the recent revolution in training techniques which has led to the rewriting of the track, field and swimming record books; and the familiar phenomenon of enterprising businessmen preying on a gullible public.

These streamlined exercises include passive massage programs, manipulation of the limbs, vibrators and vibration tables; isometric exercises; and short-duration routines which consist of a few daily exercises.

Knowing what you now know about the real nature of physical fitness, you can see why none of these programs are of any significant value.

Passive programs may help to stimulate the circulation and bring some relief from nervous tension, but they obviously can't do much to improve your motor fitness.

Isometric exercises are designed to increase muscular strength by balancing opposing muscle forces against each other, and they are useful as supplements to a general training program. But muscular strength alone does not constitute physical fitness, as we have repeatedly pointed out.

The programs which come closest to being valuable are useless because of the very factor which makes them so appealing—their brevity. Because of their brevity they are no significant help by any standard of measurement: they do not reduce fatty tissue; they do not improve motor fitness; and they rarely improve muscular strength significantly.

CALORIES.   Because of popular interest in calories, most people realize that the accumulation of fat occurs when caloric intake is greater than caloric output, and the excess is stored in the form of fatty tissue, especially if the metabolic rate is low.

The average sedentary middle-aged man absorbs about 4,000 calories in the course of a usual day. During the same period, his basal metabolism burns about 1,560 calories and his ordinary daily activity uses up another 2,000 (assuming he is even moderately active). This makes a total of 3,560 calories consumed in a day, which means that he has consumed about 440 more calories than he has burned. These calories get stored as fat. In order for this individual to lose weight by means of an exercise program he would have to burn more than 440 calories during the time that he exercised each day.

According to a series of tests which we performed at the Research Center the maximum expenditure of calories in any one of the eleven-minute exercise levels of a popular short-duration program was 110.07—far below the necessary level of energy expenditure. The average of the six levels was an expenditure of only about 85 calories.

Testing and retesting a subject who was using a short-duration program over a period of time, in order to measure any signs of improvement in any area, we found that over-all fat reduction was virtually insignificant, that there was little improvement in muscular endurance, strength and blood pressure, and that the subject was not able to improve his score on any of our standard tests, including the eighteen-item motor-fitness test.

In still another test we compared the motor-fitness abilities of groups of people with various exercise habits with a group that relied on short-duration programs for exercise, and found that the latter group scored comparatively low on the scale.

As we said, the real shortcoming of most short-duration exercise programs is the shortness of their duration. If you were to take one such program and extend it from eleven minutes to an hour, it would be reasonably effective; caloric expenditure would be multiplied approximately sixfold. But more important, it would promote cardiovascular fitness and raise the metabolic rate by even more than a multiple of six.

The real value of any exercise program lies in making a sustained effort, in pushing oneself up to and beyond the level of initial fatigue. Exercising for ten to fifteen minutes is a waste of time, since one cannot develop the reserves that lie *beyond* the point of initial fatigue if one barely *approaches* the point of fatigue.

But even extending a short-duration program to an hour does not come close to the kind of calorie expenditure that other forms of exercise produce. In their book, *Physiology of Exercise,* Laurence E. Morehouse and Augustus T. Miller list the calorie expenditure that various activities involve. At one end of the scale is sleeping, which burns 70 calories an hour. An hour of the more vigorous exercises of a typical short-duration program would bring about an expenditure of roughly 500 calories. Mountain climbing requires 600; parallel-bar work, 710; running on a slightly graded motor-driven treadmill at 7 mph, 950; rowing at 12 mph, 1,500; swimming the crawl at 2.2 mph, 1,600; and hard flat running at 12 mph, 2,330.

From these statistics you might draw the conclusion that the simple solution to achieving radical weight reduction is an hour of hard running. Unfortunately, the expenditure of 2,330 calories in an hour is a theoretical statistic. Research at the Harvard Fatigue Laboratory, the Carnegie Institution in Washington, and in various performance laboratories at Illinois, UCLA, Oregon, Johns Hopkins, and Minnesota Universities indicates that the average young man can exercise enough to burn a maximum of 700 calories per hour, while a man of forty-five can only burn about 350, unless exceptionally well trained.

So in addition to reducing fat by burning calories, another function of a good exercise program should be to increase a person's capacity to burn up calories.

Thus, it should be perfectly clear why a good one-hour-a-day exercise program is preferable to a short-duration program: in addition to helping you to burn calories, it will increase your power to expend more calories the longer you exercise. In fact, physical training on a progressive basis has been shown to increase working capacity by two to four times within a period of six months to a year.

The program of exercises that will be presented later in this section is tailor-made to fit the needs of any person who wants to get in shape or stay in shape. It has been carefully tested in our laboratories and has proved to be more efficient and effective in burning calories, increasing the power to burn calories, raising the metabolism, strengthening the heart, keeping a high volume of blood flowing, and creating a demand by the muscles for more oxygen and nutrients than any other known form of exercise.

This program is not tricky, or streamlined, or esoteric . . . or easy. It requires determination, drive and patience. But, as we at the Center have proved in hundreds of hours of tests, and as I have tried to make clear to you, this is the only real and efficient way to physical fitness.

11. Preparing to Exercise

Before you begin an active program, there are a number of things you should do to prepare yourself. The following are some items of general advice, as well as answers to some questions you may have in mind:

ARE YOU PHYSICALLY SOUND?   Before you do anything in the way of exercise, you should make sure that your body is physically sound. At the Center, we take a thorough health history and perform a medical examination on everyone who enters our program. If you are over thirty, you should get a complete examination from your own doctor before you tackle a strenuous exercise program, to determine such matters as pulse rate, blood pressure, heart, kidney and blood-vessel function and so on. Your doctor may uncover some physical defect which will affect how much and what form of exercise is right for you. He may be able to clear up any problems you may have, or he may decide to work out a program to fit your individual needs. In general, however, the likelihood is that he'll find you physically sound and capable of undertaking our program. Even if you find yourself perfectly fit, you will not have wasted your time, for the results of your doctor's tests will provide you with information which you'll be able to use as a measuring stick of your improvement.

THE RIGHT TIMES TO EXERCISE.   The best time to exercise is whenever you can find the time. The only periods we do not recommend are just after meals and right after waking up in the morning.

If you're like most people we have tested at the Center, you'll be able to work out either during your lunch hour or just after work. It may require will power to stop at your local "Y" or athletic club during or after a hard day of work, but there are immediate, as well as long-run, benefits.

Many people who exercise during lunch hours report that they work more efficiently during the afternoon. And because of the time given over to exercise they eat lighter lunches—a habit that's all to the good.

A workout after office hours—far from leaving you yawning, as you might expect—should leave you feeling refreshed and lively, ready for an evening of activity.

If you can't find the time earlier in the day, try exercising before you go to bed at night. There's no finer preparation for a good night's sleep. A warm bath after the exercise will leave you feeling relaxed.

HOW OFTEN SHOULD YOU EXERCISE?   One of the marvels of physical training is the increasing speed with which the body adapts itself to strenuous physical exercise. For instance, you may find certain exercises agonizing during the first week or two, but if you keep doing them you'll find they become easier and easier.

As a rule, we advise the average untrained person to limit himself to two to three workouts a week during the first month of the program. He can then step this rate up to three to four workouts a week during the second month, and five to six a week thereafter. Exercising on weekends only is better than not exercising at all, but we've never found it sufficient to maintain a good level of fitness.

THE RIGHT PLACE TO EXERCISE.   Obviously, the ideal place to exercise is wherever the best facilities are available. Your local athletic club or "Y" can provide you with equipment, locker rooms, steam rooms, showers and, perhaps most important, an atmosphere that is conducive to physical activity.

But if for some reason these facilities are not available to you, there is no reason why you can't make use of your own home. Many endurance exercises require no special environment. These include twisting, stretching, bending, flexing the arms, push-ups, sit-ups, squat jumps, and an infinite variety of others—enough indeed to make it possible for you to undertake a full program using your own resources. Lack of special equipment or facilities is no cause for despair or excuse not to exercise.

Another excellent place to work out is in the water, for swimming is one of the best ways to exercise. The easy, rhythmic movements of swimming are the best stimulants to an active flow of blood. In the water, the body is buoyed up so that there is almost no weight to inhibit your movement, and the water itself tones up the body generally and stimulates the metabolism.

Even if you don't have your own swimming pool, or access to a neighbor's pool, it is easy for practically anyone to find a place to swim.

THE PROPER CLOTHES TO WEAR.   No matter where or under what conditions you are exercising, you will want to wear close-fitting, brief clothing which allows you freedom of movement. Your clothing should always be clean, especially your underwear and socks. Clean clothing will absorb perspiration more readily, and it prevents skin irritation and fungus infection.

For indoor work, you should wear regular gym trunks and a T-shirt, or, if you are a woman, a leotard. In the privacy of your home, underwear is perfectly adequate. For outdoor work in the spring and summer, wear shorts and a T-shirt, or a leotard. Keep a jacket or sweat shirt handy to put on after exercising. For fall and early winter, wear sweat pants or loose-fitting slacks. When the weather gets colder (yes, you should still be exercising), just add a pair of light-weight cotton, or cotton and wool, long underwear lowers, a sweat shirt or sweater and a light-weight outer jacket.

What you wear on your feet is also important. Your shoes should fit well and they should make you feel bouncier and more agile. Wear athletic socks—one heavy pair of woolens with a light pair of cottons underneath, or two light pairs.

MUSCLE SORENESS.   Some muscle soreness should be expected with any conditioning program, especially in the early stages. Still, there are a few precautionary measures you can take to keep muscle soreness to a minimum.

At the early stages, it is a good idea to exercise only until you are moderately out of breath. Then give yourself a change of pace by spending one to two minutes breathing deeply and stretching. (For example, place your hands behind your neck and stretch your elbows backward while inhaling deeply. Then exhale and relax. Or rise on your toes and stretch your arms up overhead while taking a deep breath; then exhale and relax.) This period of breathing and stretching will allow you to recuperate, so that you can safely wind up your workout with a fairly strenuous program.

Swimming is helpful after hard exercise, especially if you make sure to shake out the joints of your arms and legs.

It will also help you avoid soreness if you will try not to exercise the same muscle group twice in succession in a very difficult tension exercise, such as push-ups, chinning the bar, or any one of a number of exercises described in the following chapters. After exercising a certain muscle group, always try to allow it time to recover before exercising it again.

To repeat, some muscle soreness is inevitable and not really cause for great concern. After all, you probably haven't used certain muscles for a long time. However, if serious pain does develop and persist, you should consult your physician. Probably you will find that you have ruptured some muscle fibers—a common occurrence, even among great athletes, and one that heals quickly.

BATHING.   Unless you intend to do your exercising before going to bed (in which case you should stick to warm showers or baths), you will find it stimulating and beneficial to take a cold shower or bath when you finish. If you find it a bit uncomfortable at first, try approaching it gradually by starting with lukewarm water and making it colder gradually. After a while, you'll find it easy to step right into an icy shower. In fact, it becomes a very pleasant sensation. And it will help your circulation and muscle tone.

12. Advice for Women

If you are a woman you may have glanced at the table of contents and turned to this chapter first. You may now be wondering why this special chapter for women appears so far on in the book, and you may suspect that its location is an indication that this book is really for men.

COMMON PROBLEMS OF MEN AND WOMEN.   Nothing could be further from the truth. Our program for physical fitness applies equally to men and women. In fact, in some respects the message of this book applies even more to women than it does to men. That is why we have waited until now to devote special attention to women.

One point of this book is to discredit the popular notion that physical fitness is a matter of appearance, that health begins on the surface. This notion is popular in the United States; it may very well be more popular among women than men.

Women, as a rule, are more conscious of their physical beings than men are. They are more sensitive to the aging process, and naturally want to hold on to their youthful beauty and vigor, and retain a good figure and an attractive complexion. For these reasons, they will go to greater efforts to help themselves than most men will.

But in this country women are poorly educated in the scientific facts of physical fitness. They are bombarded by advertising and publicity urging them to buy this facial cream for their complexions, to use that vibrating machine to tighten up slack muscles, to try such-and-such a new diet to remove unwanted fat. The trouble is that these alleged remedies are often costly, usually ineffective, and sometimes even dangerous.

EXPERIMENTAL WORK WITH WOMEN.   As an illustration, I recall one woman who appeared at the Center and asked to be admitted to a women's experimental fitness program that we were then working with. She was a forty-year-old socialite who spent most of her time planning parties and benefits and very little time in physically demanding activity.

In the process of putting her through a series of introductory tests, we discovered that she was almost helpless physically; she was unable to pass a single one of our eighteen basic motor fitness tests. She had the equivalent of only one and one-half pounds of strength per pound of body weight, she was extremely short-winded and she had very little endurance.

When we explained the results of the tests to her, she expressed great surprise and produced bills she had paid for massages, mud-baths, manipulations and "health treatments" (colonic purging) amounting to nearly nine thousand dollars in three years. All we could say was that she had received a pretty poor return for her money.

The fact of the matter is that women require the same kind of training program as men. With only slight variations (which will be noted), the same exercises are equally useful. But before women can throw themselves wholeheartedly into a strenuous program, they must be convinced that youthful vigor and beauty, good complexion, and a trim but sturdy body can come only from inside. They should feel no doubt that vigorous physical exercise will do more for any woman than all the patent nostrums combined.

The woman who is really concerned about her physical well-being must overcome the erroneous psychological attitude that there is something unfeminine about exercising the muscles. She must accept the fact that there is simply no adequate substitute for walking, running, swimming and gymnastic exercises—no matter what the glamor advertisements may say.

Some time ago, a woman came to us because she wanted to lose weight. To some extent she had accepted the fact that it was going to take more than electric vibrators and low-calorie diets to accomplish her objective, but she continued to shy away from what she regarded as masculine activities. When we explained some of our programs to her, she chose to work with an exercycle, a relatively passive device designed to exercise the muscles by flexing the legs and the torso. After six months of work which was gradually increased until she was riding two hours each day, she found that she had lost no weight at all. She was terribly disappointed, but since it was an experimental program we encouraged her to continue. When she finally gave up in despair, we determined that it took nearly 2500 hours of work on the contraption to reduce one pound of fat.

The program that I mentioned was set up to determine if the same remarkable results which had occurred with some five hundred men who had taken the course could also be obtained with women.

The age range of the women who participated ran from twenty-four to fifty-five years old. The youngest of the group, a housewife, was able to pass only 10 of the 18 motor fitness tests at the outset. At the end of the course, she passed 15. Another member of the group, aged thirty-seven, was an associate professor of home economics who took our course on the advice of her physician. As a result of her sedentary pattern of living, her first series of tests showed that she had very poor muscle tone and that her energy reserves were very low. When she started the course, she could pass only 2 of the 18 tests. At the end of the program she felt so greatly improved, both physically and mentally, that she recommended a planned-exercise program for all her students.

SOME FINDINGS.   A number of pertinent points emerged from the over-all results of our program. Almost all of the women who participated were primarily interested in getting rid of excess fat and regaining their youthful figures. The most important thing that they learned was that losing weight is only a small part of the process. One woman, for instance, lost only nine pounds, yet the improvement in her physical proportions was more dramatic than the loss of weight would indicate. What had happened was that at the same time she shed fat she gained in muscle weight, *not as the result of increased muscle size but from increased muscular density.* In addition to becoming slimmer, her figure became firmer and more flexible—a much more desirable result than mere cutting down on caloric intake would have achieved.

By setting up a control group which simply dieted and lost weight, we found that weight loss without muscle development led to a poorer performance on the fitness tests. A youthful figure isn't worth much without a youthful vitality to go with it.

We also found that in some cases women actually gained weight and still improved their measurements, not to mention their general sense of well-being.

The message that emerges from these results is clear: If women truly wish to gain the youthful appearance and vigor that they spend so much time and money trying to achieve, they must get rid of the common prejudice against supposedly "unfeminine activity." They must learn to practice the principles that apply in our training of championship swimmers, gymnasts and runners. They must accept the notion of using medicine balls, pulley weights and rowing machines; of doing exercises that develop the chest and shoulder muscles. After all, I seriously doubt if any woman could have serious complaints about having the figure that some of the members of the United States women's Olympic team have.

HOW EXERCISE BENEFITS WOMEN ESPECIALLY.   There are even distinct ways in which an intensive training program will benefit you as a woman. Frequently, it will work as an antidote to the fatigue and tension that both the housewife and the professional woman are heir to. Lack of total body movement, trying to do more than there is time for, and poor circulation are all conditions that are associated with inner tension and anxiety in adults. A day in the outdoors can be wonderfully relaxing. Rhythmical exercise, like walking, swimming, bicycling and so on, can have a similar effect.

Just getting away from disorder and confusion is part of the therapy. A daily routine of physical workouts will become something that you will look forward to as a pleasant oasis in a hectic schedule.

Women often find that interest in exercise and physical fitness brings them closer to their husbands or boy friends. A willingness to ignore the hardships of the outdoors, to try such activities as horseback riding, shooting, camping out, skiing and fishing can bring you to a common ground with many men, as well as benefit your health and state of mind.

Finally, and perhaps most important, exercise can help to relieve the discomfort that many women experience during their menstrual periods. There have been many studies in sport-medical literature showing that women athletes are able to compete comfortably during their periods and that exertion actually eases their discomfort. Exercise has the effect of keeping body heat up, which is especially desirable during menstruation, when blood congests in the uterus. If a woman exercises to the point where she perspires moderately, blood will circulate more freely throughout her body. And the tilting of the pelvis in stretching movements which flatten the lower back helps to relieve the tensions, the congestion of blood and the consequent discomfort in critical regions.

So, if you are a woman you can follow the advice and the program given in this book just as if it had been written especially for you. In most cases, if a particular exercise is not suitable for women, an appropriate adaptation is suggested. In every case, you will understand the principle that lies behind our suggestions and be able to adapt it to your own particular situation. All it takes is a little imagination and a good dose of will power.

13. A Home Exercise Program

FIRST MONTH: LOW–GEAR EXERCISE

The exercise program that is presented in the following chapters is an informal one, designed so that you can take it on your own, in your own home. It differs from the program that is presented in Part Two of this book in that it is simpler, shorter, puts less emphasis on special gymnasium equipment and is designed for people who are not in extremely poor condition.

The following program is divided into three general stages, which we call low gear, middle gear and high gear. Each of these stage increases in difficulty so that you can work your way into an intensive program gradually. This means that you need not coast and take it easy at the early stages; you can apply yourself vigorously from the start, with the knowledge that the exercises won't make too great demands on your body.

Each daily exercise period is divided into two phases: a thirty-minute period of warm-up exercises which are intended to get the blood flowing and build up respiration and body heat, and a thirty-minute period of endurance exercises designed to build stamina and increase the efficiency of the heart action.

PHASE ONE
10 Low-Gear
Exercises

You should allot five minutes to each exercise or group of exercises. After each five-minute exercise period you should rest, stretch, and take ten full breaths.

It is very important to get into the habit of breathing deeply and continually both during and between exercises. If you succumb to the natural tendency to hold your breath while exerting yourself you will tire more quickly from the lack of oxygen supply to your muscles.

EXERCISE ONE.   As a rule, the upper body and shoulders are not used to their full potential. You should concentrate particularly hard on the exercises that will build up this segment of the body.

1. BODY SEGMENT AND PRINCIPAL MUSCLE GROUPS USED

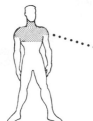

NECK, SHOULDERS,
UPPER BACK AND CHEST,
NECK AND SHOULDER RETRACTORS,
ARM ELEVATORS AND CHEST ELEVATORS

1. Stand upright with your feet slightly apart. Flex your arms and bring your fists sharply up to your chest. Swing your arms down, forward, then up and over head, as far back as possible; look up, raise your chest and stretch; then swing your arms back to original position. Repeat the exercise rhythmically again and again. With each upward swing of the arms take a deep breath, fill your lungs with air, and hold your breath a few seconds while looking up and stretching your chest.

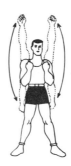

EXERCISE TWO.   As a result of sedentary living, a number of things tend to go wrong with your body. The lower back muscles weaken, sometimes causing dull ache and even severe pain; the circulation in this area is apt to become inadequate; the muscles of the buttocks tend to soften and lose their tone. These tendencies can be offset with the proper exercises.

As a result of these tendencies the pelvis tilts forward and downward, causing a protuberant stomach and a hollow back, or what posture teachers refer to as an S-curve. You can correct this tendency by consciously tilting the pelvis upward by tensing the buttock muscles. It will help you to do this if you will place your back against a wall or lie with your back on the floor.

2. BODY SEGMENT AND PRINCIPAL MUSCLE GROUPS USED

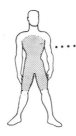

BACK REGION,
BUTTOCKS AND UPPER LEGS,
HAMSTRINGS,
GLUTEI AND SACROSPINALIS

2. Lie on your stomach, with your hands
tucked under your thighs, your back arched
and your chest and head off the floor. Now
flutter-kick continuously, with the legs 8 to
10 inches apart, moving your legs from the
hips with a slight bend at the knees, one
leg going up while the other is going down,
and vice-versa, but never touching the floor.
Breathe regularly and deeply while doing
this exercise.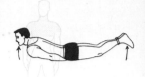

EXERCISES THREE AND FOUR.   Poor condition of the abdominal muscles, coupled with flaccid leg veins, results in pooling of the blood in
the lower abdomen and legs both while the individual is sitting and
standing. We refer to this condition as "pot belly." In addition to doing
the following two exercises, you can counteract the development of a
pot belly by rhythmical contraction of the abdominal muscles in leg-
lifts and sit-ups, while simultaneously slapping the abdominal wall.
Cold bathing will also help to stimulate the circulation and improve
the tone of the muscles.

3. & 4. BODY SEGMENT AND PRINCIPAL MUSCLE GROUPS USED

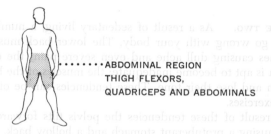

•••••••ABDOMINAL REGION
THIGH FLEXORS,
QUADRICEPS AND ABDOMINALS

3. Assume a sitting position, with your legs
outstretched, your hands on your hips or on
the floor at the hips. Pull your left knee to
your chest, then as you straighten this leg,
pull your right knee to your chest. Alter-
nate and continue until you are tired.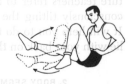

4. Get down on your hands and knees. Take a
deep breath, suck in your abdomen toward
the spine and hold for a few seconds. Then
lower your body to the floor, breathe out
fully, and stretch two or three times,
breathing out as fully as possible. Repeat.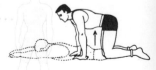

EXERCISE FIVE.   Other casualties of the sedentary existence are the waist and the sides of the body, particularly the muscles that are used in bending the body sideways to the right or to the left and in all twisting movements of the trunk upon the pelvis.

5. BODY SEGMENT AND PRINCIPAL MUSCLE GROUPS USED

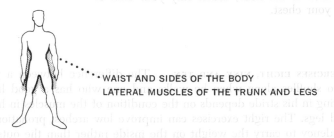

WAIST AND SIDES OF THE BODY
LATERAL MUSCLES OF THE TRUNK AND LEGS

5. Lying full length, with the right side of your body on the floor, and your head resting on your hand, whip your left leg up and down in rapid motion 12 inches off the floor 50 times. Repeat exercise with left side of your body on the floor, raising your right leg 50 times.

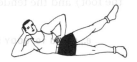

EXERCISES SIX AND SEVEN.   These exercises concentrate once more on the upper part of the body—the part that suffers particularly as a result of the lack of wood-chopping and water-hauling in modern life.

6. and 7. BODY SEGMENT AND PRINCIPAL MUSCLE GROUPS USED

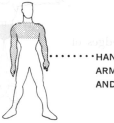

HANDS, ARMS AND SHOULDERS
ARM EXTENSORS AND FLEXORS
AND ENTIRE SHOULDER GIRDLE

6. Lying on your back, with your legs outstretched, lift and bend one leg, grasp the knee with fingers laced, and, while resisting with the hip muscle, pull your knee toward your chest. Then repeat the exercise with the other knee. Continue, alternating first one knee, then the other, pulling hard several times on each.

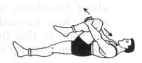

7. Lie full length on the floor with chest down, legs outstretched, knees stiff. Then, resting your weight on both hands, which should be placed directly under your shoulders, and with your back straight, do 10 full-length push-ups. Avoid touching your abdomen to the floor; touch only your chin or your chest.

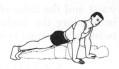

EXERCISES EIGHT, NINE AND TEN.   The difference between a person who shuffles along when he walks and one who has a good healthy spring in his stride depends on the condition of the muscles in his feet and legs. The right exercises can improve low arches, pronation (the tendency to carry the weight on the inside rather than the outside of the foot) and the tendency to bend the big toe inward.

8., 9. and 10. BODY SEGMENT AND PRINCIPAL MUSCLE GROUPS USED

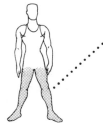

•FEET, LEGS AND ANKLES
ARCH SUPPORTERS, FOOT SUPINATORS,
FOOT EXTENSORS, LEG EXTENSORS
AND THIGH EXTENSORS

8. Walk in a circle on the outside edges of the feet.

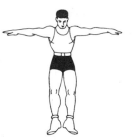

9. Facing the wall, with your feet placed about two-thirds of your body's length away, lean forward with your hands on the wall, so that the wall is holding you up. Then push up and down on your toes.

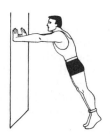

10. Assume the push-up position (see Exercise 7), point your toes in so that your weight rests on your insteps, and bounce the weight of your body on your ankles. You will feel the tension in your calves and ankle joints.

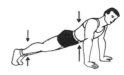

Presumably, you have now been exercising for thirty minutes. You have taken intervals between exercises to rest, stretch, and breathe deeply. You are now ready to move into phase two of the Low-Gear Program.

PHASE TWO
Endurance
Exercises

Actually, your activity during the second thirty-minute period of your daily exercise should consist of one activity—one that uses various muscle groups and requires considerable expenditure of energy.

One good example of this type of exercise is simple walking, only you should walk with long strides, take continual deep breaths, and swing your arms vigorously. Another good way to spend this thirty-minute period is swimming, using various strokes.

To start out, try walking one mile. Remember to exaggerate the shoulder, arm and hip movements in order to get the maximum good from the exercise. As you progress, try working the distance you cover up to two and then three miles.

If time and opportunity exists, you can substitute any number of other activities, as long as they are ones that require *continual* movement that you can keep up. Such activities might include rowing a boat, riding a bicycle, playing handball, squash, tennis or badminton, swimming, skating, skiing and dancing. As I have emphasized, the most important thing is that you keep these exercises up every day.

Here is what your weekly schedule might be:
Thirty minutes of exercises and
MONDAY—Walk a mile or more at a good clip,
TUESDAY—Swim a variety of strokes, a quarter mile or more,
WEDNESDAY—Shovel your sidewalk, rake leaves, or cut grass,
THURSDAY—Go square dancing, or go to a gym and work out on some apparatus like a rowing machine or a treadmill,

FRIDAY—Ride a bicycle 3 to 5 miles,
SATURDAY—Play tennis, handball or badminton,
SUNDAY—Take an hour walk.

14. Proper Dieting

Now that you are launched into your routine of exercise, let's take this interval to discuss your eating habits.

Every year dozens of books are published containing endless advice on the subject of what the human animal should eat and drink. Some of these books contain a great deal of sense, while others are filled with nonsense. Indeed, there's a lot to be said on the subject.

We don't intend to say a great deal. Obviously, we believe that consideration of the food you eat should be subordinated to the amount of exercise you take, or we would have discussed dieting earlier. Nevertheless, there are some points that should be made.

In order to get into the subject of dieting, let's backtrack a moment and review some fundamentals. As almost everyone knows, when a person consumes food he consumes calories. A calorie is an arbitrary unit of measure which stands for the amount of heat required to raise the temperature of one kilogram of water by one degree centigrade. When the term calorie is used as a unit in expressing the heat-producing or energy-producing value of food, it simply refers to the amount of energy potentially expendable in muscular work or other bodily activities. In plainer language, if you eat a tablespoonful of honey, which contains about 100 calories, you consume enough potential energy to raise the heat of one kilogram of water by 100 degrees centigrade.

Obviously, a person doesn't expend energy by heating water. But he can expend energy that can be *measured* in caloric value. If you consume 100 calories and then expend energy that is equal to 100 calories, your metabolism is balanced. For a normal person, it is ideal to consume and expend the same number of calories.

Unfortunately, for reasons we have gone into elsewhere, the average person in contemporary society tends to take in more calories than he gets rid of. Generally speaking, calories that are consumed and not expended are stored in the body in the form of fat.

Now, there are two ways that a person can alter the balance between calories consumed and calories expended: one is to *consume fewer* calories, and the other is to *expend more* calories. It follows, in theory, that if a person burns up more calories than he consumes, he is going to have to draw on his storage supply. In actuality, this works; both not eating and exercising more are effective ways to reduce fat and lose weight.

DIETING WITHOUT EXERCISE.   On the face of it, it might seem that the easy way to lose weight is to cut down on the amount you eat —to go on a "crash diet," as the expression goes. However, there are a number of drawbacks to this approach—enough indeed, to make it definitely not recommended by the majority of medical experts.

For one thing, consuming more calories than you burn is not the only way to build up fat. Muscle tissue that is not used may turn into fat. You can see that the result of dieting without exercising will be a thin weak person rather than a fat weak person. The former is hardly an improvement over the latter. The point is that, although it may improve appearances somewhat, losing weight just isn't a very important part of getting fit.

In actuality, crash diets are extremely unhealthy. They put more of a negative strain on the body than carrying excess fat does. Crash diets lower the resistance and leave the individual prone to disease, fatigue, unnatural aging, and other harmful effects.

Even diets which stress certain types of food are inadequate and frequently harmful. A rice-fruit diet, for instance, lacks the necessary amino acids, minerals and certain enzymes and vita-mins. Other popular regimens, like the banana diet and the high-protein—low-fat diet, have their drawbacks too. Except in extraor-dinary cases where a physician makes a special recommendation, it is best to consider dieting as harmful as overeating.

You can't put your body in shape by starving it. To cut down on food intake while you are not exercising leads to loss of energy, loss of muscle tone, poor endurance and loss of the supply of reserves needed for activities like sports, work and even sex life.

A good illustration of the point I am trying to make is the case of a woman who asked to join our experimental fitness program for women. For ten years she had succeeded in keeping her weight down by careful dieting. Nevertheless, she did not feel well and after a thorough medical checkup her doctor pronounced her unfit. She complained of fatigue, constipation, headaches and various internal disorders. Finally, she realized she had wasted a great deal of time, money and will power treating her problem superficially. What she needed was not a food diet but a steady dose of exercise.

EXERCISING WITHOUT DIETING.   If you must go to extremes, you will be better off exercising and eating as much as you like. All indications are that activity neutralizes the bad effects of overeating and consuming unhealthy foods. For instance, a study performed in Finland showed that lumbermen who drink heavily are able to escape with few or no adverse effects, as long as they continue to work. Similarly, professional athletes seem to be able to ignore dieting without being slowed up. And dietary experiments indicate that as long as the individual is engaged in physical labor, a high cholesterol consumption does not cause a high cholesterol blood level or high blood pressure.

Besides expending calories, physical training benefits your eating habits by making it possible for you to get more out of the food you eat. By improving the circulation, physical training makes it possible for nutritive ingredients in the food you eat to be carried to all the cells of the body. By contrast, where circulation is poor, parts of the body can literally be starved, so that certain cells and tissues die.

Paradoxically, a part of the body may be fat and still be starved. In areas where fat is concentrated, large quantities of blood become trapped, causing sluggish circulation and depriving adjacent areas of blood and an adequate supply of oxygen and nutritive elements.

Actually, consideration of the different methods of keeping

weight and fatty deposits reduced is academic, because weight is really a very poor guide to fitness in most cases. True morphological patterns of body types cannot be altered greatly. In other words, some people are going to remain on the chubby side no matter how much they exercise. All that you can really control is what is referred to as "transient fat." This is best controlled by exercise. Dieting alone cannot reduce transient fat without causing loss of fitness, strength and endurance.

EATING SENSIBLY.   Even though we recommend exercise over dieting, it is wise to be somewhat sensible in deciding what to eat. After all, why not get maximum mileage out of your fitness program when all it takes is a little extra self-control.

As a general rule, it is a good idea to cut down on foods with high caloric content and comparatively little nutritive value. It will be especially helpful if you avoid sugars, fats, starches, fried food and alcohol as much as possible.

Try to cut down on rich pastries and dairy food. Eat brown bread instead of white, with maybe a little less butter than usual. Try milk instead of cream in your coffee. Substitute gelatin for pie and cake. Some ice cream won't hurt you, but try leaving off the topping. Eat plenty of fresh fruit and more green and yellow vegetables. Drink plenty of milk and fruit juices.

Raisins, apples, carrots and celery should replace rich candies, cocktails, and pastry in your daily diet. You can also fortify your diet with vitamin and mineral supplements. While a physically active person can absorb extraordinary quantities of rich foods and alcohol without showing ill effects, following some of the foregoing advice will simply make it easier for you to benefit from your training program.

WHEAT GERM.   There is one particularly important addition that you can make to your diet—wheat germ and wheat germ oil. Wheat germ, sometimes called the "wonder fuel," is almost a complete food in itself. It is a rich source of high quality protein and carbohydrate, and it is well stocked with vitamin B-complex, iron, phosphorus, vitamin E and several other nutritive elements not found in abundance in other foods.

An interesting experiment conducted at our Center, involving the use of wheat germ oil as a supplementary diet, illustrates not only the value of the cereal, but also the value of exercise related to nutrition.

A group of men was progressively trained with the specific objective of increasing the men's endurance. They were periodically tested to determine their ability to ride a bicycle to the point of exhaustion and the fitness of their circulatory systems. The men improved steadily for twelve weeks, at which point the rates of their improvement began to level off. Then, after two weeks during which the men's performances remained on a plateau, wheat germ oil in fairly heavy doses was added to the diet. This was continued for six more weeks of hard training.

Usually when men are forced to continue intensive training every day for two or three weeks after they have reached a plateau in their performances, they simply go stale and begin to decline in the level of their performances. But in this case the men did not go stale; they began to improve again in the bicycle tests and in their cardiovascular tests.

At the same time, a control group which was not given the wheat germ oil but which was undergoing the same training program continued to go stale and decline in performance level.

While we have not yet succeeded in determining just what the factor in wheat germ is which seems to increase power and endurance, the conclusions that can be drawn from our experimental data is obvious. Wheat germ is helpful as a supplement to an intensive training program.

It is probably safe to conclude that the same is true of all good food—that the food you like is good for you as long as you are exercising.

15. A Home Exercise Program

SECOND MONTH: MIDDLE–GEAR EXERCISES

After you have continued with the low-gear exercises presented earlier for about a month, or until you feel thoroughly comfortable doing them, you will be ready to move on to what we call our Middle-Gear Program. The exercises in this program are designed to be somewhat more vigorous than those in the earlier program, though they should not put any undue strain on your body. They are adjusted to what we have found to be the capacity of any normal middle-aged man.

These exercises are arranged in the same order of progression as the group introduced for the first month. The same body segments and principal muscle groups are affected—only somewhat more intensely.

Again, each exercise should be allotted five minutes, with time out for a little relaxation before proceeding to the next. By relaxation, we mean *active* not *passive* relaxation: stretching, shaking out the muscles in your arms and legs and breathing deeply.

And again, the total daily exercise period should last one hour and be divided into two phases, one to work on specific muscles and the other to build up general endurance.

1. BODY SEGMENT AND PRINCIPAL MUSCLE GROUPS USED

PHASE ONE
10 Middle-Gear
Exercises

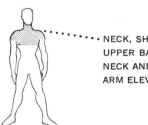
NECK, SHOULDERS,
UPPER BACK AND CHEST
NECK AND SHOULDER RETRACTORS,
ARM ELEVATORS AND CHEST ELEVATORS

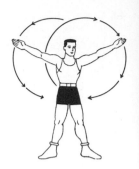

1. Standing upright, swing both your arms across the front of your body in the opposite direction from each other, up and round and down in full arm circles. Rhythmically rise on the balls of your feet with each upward swing of the arms, taking regular, full, deep breaths, inhaling as you swing the arms up, exhaling as you swing the arms down.

2. and 3. BODY SEGMENT AND PRINCIPAL MUSCLE GROUPS USED

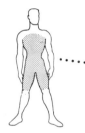

········ BACK REGION, BUTTOCKS AND UPPER LEGS
HAMSTRINGS, GLUTEI
AND SACROSPINALIS

2. Lie outstretched with your back toward the floor, supporting your body on your outstretched arms and heels. Then whip the midsection of the body up and down in rapid movement.

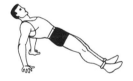

3. Lying on your stomach with your hands behind your neck, arch your body by raising your chest and legs off the floor. Do this 15 times.

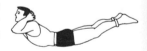

4. and 5. BODY SEGMENT AND PRINCIPAL MUSCLE GROUPS USED

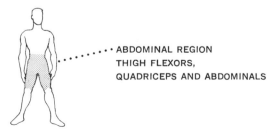

········· ABDOMINAL REGION
THIGH FLEXORS,
QUADRICEPS AND ABDOMINALS

4. Lying on your back, raise and hold both your legs outstretched, knees stiff, 4 to 5 inches off the floor. While holding this position, or while kicking your legs alternately (as if you were doing flutter kicks on your back) vigorously slap your abdominal region. Don't hold your breath; continue to breathe forcefully.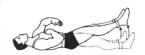

5. Assume a sitting position. Supporting yourself with your hands on the floor near your hips, tuck both knees toward your chest, then thrust the legs straight out. Do this 20 times in continuous motion.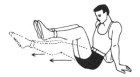

6. BODY SEGMENT AND PRINCIPAL MUSCLE GROUPS USED

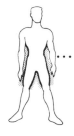

· · · · · · · WAIST AND SIDES
OF THE BODY. LATERAL MUSCLES
OF THE TRUNK AND LEGS.

6. Lying full length, with the right side of your body on the floor, whip your left leg up and down in rapid motion as high as possible off the floor 30 times. Repeat this exercise with the left side of the body on the floor, whipping your right leg off the floor 30 times.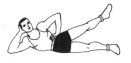

7. and 8. BODY SEGMENT AND PRINCIPAL MUSCLE GROUPS USED

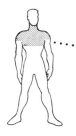

· · · · · · · HANDS, ARMS AND SHOULDERS,
ARM EXTENSORS AND FLEXORS
AND ENTIRE SHOULDER GIRDLE.

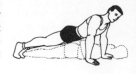

7. Lying full length on the floor, face down, legs together, hands on the floor under arm-pits with fingers pointing straight ahead, do 20 full-length push-ups by extending your arms, so that your weight rests on your hands and your toes.

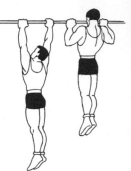

8. Chin the bar 10 times. When you grasp the chinning bar, be sure your knuckles are pointing toward your face. Start with your arms fully extended and be sure you raise your chin over the bar. (If you're working out at home, you can install a temporary bar across a doorway.)

9. and 10. BODY SEGMENT AND PRINCIPAL MUSCLE GROUPS USED

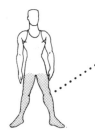

• FEET, LEGS AND ANKLES, ARCH SUPPORTERS, FOOT SUPINATORS, FOOT EXTENSORS, LEG EXTENSORS AND THIGH EXTENSORS.

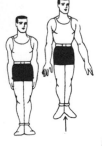

9. First hop up and down on both feet (with feet together), up to 100 times. Then change to straddle jump. (This is done by standing with feet together, jumping and landing with feet apart, and jumping and landing with feet together again.) Do this up to 100 times. Then change to scissors jump. (This is done by standing with right leg and left arm extended forward, and left leg and right arm extended backward, jumping up, and landing with arms and legs in a reversed position.) Do this up to 100 times. Finally, hop only on right foot 25 times, then only on left foot 25 times.

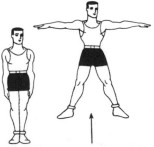

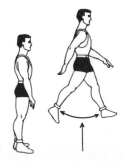

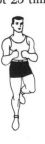

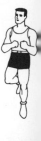

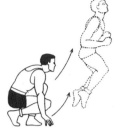

10. Do full-squat jumps, touching fingers to the floor outside your feet and springing to upright position about 4 inches in the air, and then back to a squatting position. Do continuously until you are tired.

Repeat the routine that you followed during the first month, except perform the various exercises more vigorously, if possible.

For instance, instead of walking a mile, alternate between a walk and a jog for two miles. If you are swimming, try sprinting 100 yards, then rest and breathe deeply for a minute, then sprint another 100 yards.

If the weather is bad or if you haven't the time or inclination to participate in some sport out of doors, the following exercise can be performed conveniently in your house or apartment:

PHASE TWO
Endurance
Exercises

Step up and down from a chair (or bench or stool) to the floor and back. (The chair should be 17 inches high for men; 14 inches high for women.) Lead for one minute with the left foot, then change to the right foot for a minute. Then stop, stretch, breathe deeply, and do an arm exercise or an abdominal exercise. Then repeat the routine with the chair. Increase the repetitions as the weeks go along, until you are able to perform it for a full 30 minutes.

16. A Home Exercise Program

THIRD MONTH: HIGH–GEAR EXERCISES

When you are ready to move into the High-Gear Program after two months or so, you will have reached the level of exertion that you should keep up henceforth if you wish to stay in good condition. It is a good idea to stick to your schedule pretty rigidly, for you will find that if you succumb to the temptation to skip a day or two, it is more difficult to resume exercising the following day.

These high-gear exercises are arranged in the same order of progression as the group of exercises you have been using during the two previous months. They apply to the same body segments and principal muscle groups as those you did during the first two months.

PHASE ONE
10 High-Gear
Exercises

As you did at the two previous levels of exercise, devote five minutes to each exercise, then rest and take ten full breaths as you stretch the part of your body that you just finished exercising.

1. BODY SEGMENT AND PRINCIPAL MUSCLE GROUPS USED

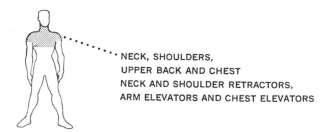

NECK, SHOULDERS,
UPPER BACK AND CHEST
NECK AND SHOULDER RETRACTORS,
ARM ELEVATORS AND CHEST ELEVATORS

1. Stand with your legs wide apart. Swing your right arm up and overhead counter-clockwise across body, then bend from the waist with knees stiff and touch your hand to the floor as far outside of the opposite foot as possible. Then whip arm back over-head, fast and hard, to original position, at the same time straightening up. All this should, of course, be one continuous move-ment. Now repeat, using left arm. Swing left arm up and overhead, bend and touch left hand to the floor as far outside of right foot as possible. While doing this exercise, suck in and blow out air forcefully, exhaling while touching the floor and inhaling while changing sides. Do exercise 15 times on each side.

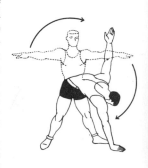

2. BODY SEGMENT AND PRINCIPAL MUSCLE GROUPS USED

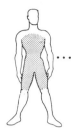 ········· BACK REGION,
BUTTOCKS AND UPPER LEGS
HAMSTRINGS, GLUTEI
AND SACROSPINALIS

2. Lie outstretched on your stomach, with your hands behind your neck. Now do the following exercise in 4 counts: (a) arch your back, so as to lift your legs and chest off the floor; (b) holding this position, extend arms fully forward; (c) return hands to neck; (d) flatten body to floor and relax one second. Repeat this whole exercise 15 times. Then lie on your back and stretch while taking very deep breaths.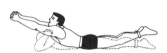

3. and 4. BODY SEGMENT AND PRINCIPAL MUSCLE GROUPS USED

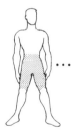 ········· ABDOMINAL REGION
THIGH FLEXORS,
QUADRICEPS AND ABDOMINALS

3. Lying on your back with your body outstretched, your legs together and your knees stiff, raise your legs to a vertical position, then slowly lower them back to the floor. Do this 20 times. Then get on your hands and knees, and stretch and breathe deeply.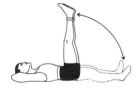

4. From the same position, in 4 counts, (a) raise your legs together 12 to 18 inches from the floor; (b) spread legs apart as far as possible; (c) return legs together; (d) lower legs to floor. Do 20 times.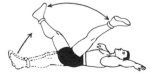

5. BODY SEGMENT AND PRINCIPAL MUSCLE GROUPS USED

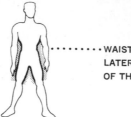

· · · · · · · · · WAIST AND SIDES OF THE BODY
LATERAL MUSCLES
OF THE TRUNK AND LEGS

5. With the right side of your body down, rigidly supported off the floor by your right foot and your extended right arm, raise your left leg to a horizontal position and lower it again to right leg. Repeat this 30 times. Then do this exercise with the left side of the body down, raising the right leg to horizontal position 30 times.

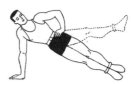

6. and 7. BODY SEGMENT AND PRINCIPAL MUSCLE GROUPS USED

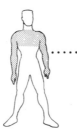

· · · · · · · · · HANDS, ARMS AND SHOULDERS
ARM EXTENSORS
AND FLEXOR AND ENTIRE
SHOULDER GIRDLE

6. Lying chest down on the floor, legs outstretched, resting your body on both hands, do full-length push-ups 20 times or more.

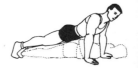

7. Chin the bar 12 times or more. When you grasp the chinning bar, be sure your knuckles are pointing toward your face. Start with your arms fully extended and be sure you raise your chin over the bar.

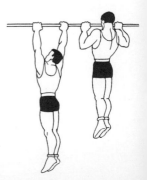

8. 9. and 10. BODY SEGMENT AND PRINCIPAL MUSCLE GROUPS USED

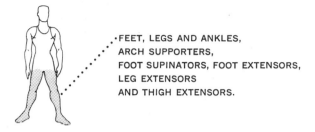

•FEET, LEGS AND ANKLES,
ARCH SUPPORTERS,
FOOT SUPINATORS, FOOT EXTENSORS,
LEG EXTENSORS
AND THIGH EXTENSORS.

8. Hop on both feet 200 times. Then do straddle hop 200 times. Then do alternate-stride hop 200 times. Next, hop on each foot continuously 50 times. Finally, do up to 50 full-squat jumps, touching fingers to floor each time and springing 4 inches off floor to upright position.

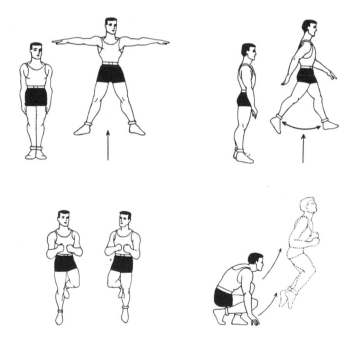

9. Breathe hard for one minute, then take 3 long, deep breaths and hold as long as possible.

10. Take, in succession, 10 long, deep breaths and hold the last one 15 seconds.

PHASE TWO
Endurance
Exercises

Once again, repeat the routines that you have developed during the two previous months, but work out more strenuous versions.

For instance, instead of walking and jogging when you do road-work, walk a mile, run a mile, walk a quarter of a mile, sprint 200 yards, and walk a half-mile each day. Then breathe deeply while stretching your chest.

Or, to develop maximum motor ability and endurance, strenuously engage in one of the following activities: swimming, cycling, rowing, bowling, skating, skiing, dancing, handball, golf or any other activity which exerts various muscles of the body, increases agility and develops endurance.

17. Where Do You Go from Here?

Now that you have completed approximately three months of exercising, you should begin to be noticing some improvement in your general condition. You might at this point take the physical fitness and motor fitness tests over again. You should notice significant improvement in your performance.

But don't expect a miracle. It takes a good six months to make a real improvement. And even then you can't expect to rest on your laurels. If you do, and return to your old habits, you'll find that all your work has been wasted.

The plain fact is that nobody ever graduates from the school of physical conditioning. You either continue working or you go downhill. You can't live on your capital; you have to live on the interest paid on the investment of continual hard work.

GENERAL GUIDELINES.   In conclusion, let's review some of the principles of a physically fit existence. These can be considered guidelines that you should follow for the rest of your life.

You should continue to promote the flow of your blood by means of rhythmic endurance exercise for at least thirty minutes a day, three days a week, in order to open up capillaries which might otherwise stay unopened, in order to strengthen the heart and improve the function of the blood vessels. As a result, your pulse rate will remain slow, the stroke volume of your heart will remain sharp and strong, and your diastolic blood pressure will remain low.

You should swim in cold water in order to maintain good muscular tone and circulatory and respiratory fitness, and to keep down nervous tension. Water pressure is important in itself, but swimming also requires rhythmic movements which are highly beneficial to blood flow. The stimulation of cool water on the skin produces a mild vaso-constriction which forces the blood inward and increases its supply to the inner organs, the glands, the heart and the nerve centers. Once you've gotten used to the mild shock of cold water you'll find swimming a calming and refreshing experience.

Bathing under ultraviolet light three times a week, fully exposed but in moderate doses, will act to lower your pulse rate and blood pressure, increase your basal metabolism, and increase the production of vitamin D in your skin.

Reduction of fried foods, heavy creams, ice cream, pie crust, cake and sugar in your diet is highly beneficial. Carbohydrates in the form of mashed, baked, or boiled potatoes and in beans and toast should not be eliminated entirely, but they should be eaten in moderation. Your diet should be supplemented with wheat germ, wheat germ oil, whole grains, natural fruits and vegetables, and skimmed milk. Wheat germ oil and vitamin B and C supplements should preferably be taken just before or after exercising.

Vitaminized yeast, sodium phosphate, and cod liver oil during the winter months are good dietary supplements. Fruit juice should be taken regularly in large quantities, in order to increase the alkaline buffering properties of the blood and also to strengthen the capillaries.

Naturally, it will help you to moderate your consumption of alcoholic beverages and eliminate tobacco entirely.

Outdoor activity, including moderate exposure to wind, sun and cold, should be part of your year-round activity. Camping out is a particularly satisfying way of exposing yourself to the elements.

Emotionally gratifying activity in reasonable proportion to work and routine will help you stay physically fit. But most of all, it is regular day-by-day exercising to the point of fatigue that will help you maintain a high level of fitness.

THE IDEAL ATTITUDE.   All of these principles must become a permanent part of your life, not a series of self-conscious habits. The following little story illustrates what we mean by a proper attitude toward physical fitness.

In 1952 we went to Europe to conduct some research at the Olympic Games in Helsinki, Finland. During a stay in England I had the opportunity to test a number of great athletes of the past and present at the Royal Free Medical College in London. Among these athletes were men like Roger Bannister, McDonald Bailey and Arthur Wint.

One day Sam Ferris, a former great in English track history, appeared before us. Sam had run second to Juan Carlos Zabala of Argentina in the 1932 Olympic marathon in Los Angeles. It was a steaming hot day and the macadam road they ran on was even hotter. Nevertheless, both Juan Carlos and Sam broke the Olympic marathon record established by the great Hannes Kolehmainen at Antwerp twelve years earlier.

After giving Sam many of the tests, I found myself deeply impressed by how good his score was. So I said, "Sam, when I find a person with scores as good as yours I always try to find out what sort of program he uses to keep fit."

"But I don't have any program," Sam replied. "I gave up training years ago."

We continued with the tests, and as we came to the harder ones, Sam's scores got better and better. Again I said, "Sam, you must tell me how you keep so fit." And still he denied having any formula, program or secret.

On a hunch, I asked Sam how far he lived from his work. He said, "About sixteen miles," and then added, "I ride to work on a bicycle."

"You ride to work and back on a bicycle?" I exclaimed.

"Yes," he said. "Five days a week."

Thirty-two miles a day; one hundred and sixty miles a week! And Sam thought he had given up exercising.

"Oh," he said. "I don't consider that exercise. I gave up running years ago; that was real exercise."

Sam Ferris had the sort of standard of fitness that I wish we could instill in everyone. He maintained it with steady, rhythmical exercise, day in and day out. And he showed the results.

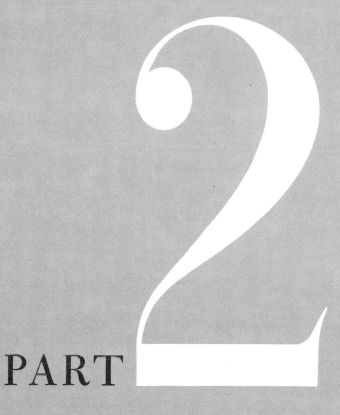

PART **2**

*A Practical Program
for
Physical Fitness*

General Introduction

The following series of twenty-two lessons has been developed as the result of years of practical work with adult men and women. The lessons make up a course that is the best and most efficient method we know for working a person into top physical condition, no matter how badly his (or her) condition may have deteriorated over the years.

Unlike the program that was presented in Part One of this book, the following course is primarily intended to be taken as a formal class, complete with equipment and instructor. However, if you do not have either the time or the means to devote to a formal class, the course will still prove useful to you. After seeing one or two demonstrations by a trained instructor, and with a little imagination, discretion and self-discipline, you can adapt it for your personal convenience and use it as a conditioning program in your own home and in your own time. The course includes a large variety of exercises, and those that require special equipment can be replaced by others which do not and which will do just as well.

Nevertheless, there are distinct advantages to working with a formal class. An experienced instructor can demonstrate exactly how the exercises are executed; he can organize and control the progress of the class; he can set the proper pace; and he can give individual help and advice when and where it is needed. Furthermore, working in a group provides an atmosphere of mutual effort and competition that provides a psychological lift and helps you to drive yourself faster and longer. Just as an infantry soldier finds that he can march farther with seemingly less effort when he is marching in formation, you will find it easier to work with others around you to a clear and insistent cadence.

HOW TO JOIN A CLASS.   The course that is outlined in the following chapter can be taken formally in most YMCAs, YMHAs, schools, colleges and universities, community recreation centers and athletic clubs. If you are unable to find a course being offered, you can help organize one through your own local community organization. All you need are the facilities available in any school or community gymnasium and a qualified physical education instructor. You should have no trouble finding people like yourself who are eager to organize a class, for the need for such training has become so obvious among large numbers of sedentary people that more and more people are looking for solutions to their exercise problems.

HOW THE COURSE IS ORGANIZED.   The course is divided into twenty-two lessons, which should be completed in from six to nine months, depending on the age and physical condition of the members of the class. These factors need not necessarily be uniform, since the lessons are organized to allow the individual members to progress at their own pace and according to their own needs.

The course progresses in difficulty from low gear to middle gear to high gear. Low-gear work is meant to develop flexibility, and consists of rhythmical endurance exercises at a slow pace, with emphasis on deep breathing timed properly with the exercises. The minimum objective is thirty minutes of continuous exercises three days per week.

Middle-gear work consists of moderately hard exercises done faster and for longer periods. The minimum objective is one hour of continuous, stepped-up exercise, four days per week. You should devote one day a week to two hours of longer, harder work.

High-gear work consists of hard exercise at least three days per week, and a minimum of five ninety-minute exercise periods a week. By this stage in the course you will have progressively worked up to performing highly taxing exercises, at high speeds, over long periods of time. You will also find yourself in first-rate physical condition.

THE LESSONS.   The individual lessons are, as a rule, divided into four major sections: (1) A brief introduction discussing some aspect of the lesson or the course which should either be read by you or delivered in the form of a talk by the instructor; (2) a period of warm-up exercises designed to build up body heat, circulation and respiration, and to protect your muscles and joints from strain by reducing their resistance; (3) the main body of the lesson, consisting of various kinds of relatively strenuous exercises; and (4) a tapering-off, or recovery, period, which emphasizes deep breathing, stretching, massage and rest.

It should be understood that all of these lessons have been tested on ordinary, untrained adults without adverse effects. While you may feel that the workouts are too long, remember that caloric expenditure is greater in proportion to the time spent. That is why workouts lasting thirty minutes or longer are more effective than those lasting only ten or fifteen minutes.

Once the individual workout begins, the emphasis should be on continuous and progressive build-up of speed and exertion. The important thing is not so much to perform the exercises in a precise and exactly correct way as to develop a continuous, nonstop routine. That is why actvities which require sporadic bursts of energy, like softball, basketball and tennis are not truly effective for physical conditioning.

THE EXERCISES.   The many different exercises presented in this course are designed to exert all the major parts of your body, in a variety of combinations and for different purposes. Each exercise should also be performed at three levels of intensity: low-gear, middle-gear, and high-gear. At each different stage of the course a different level of exertion should of emphasized. For instance, at the low-gear level each exercise should be performed slowly and deliberately, with the emphasis on learning and properly timed breathing. At the middle-gear level, each exercise should be performed first slowly, then faster, then at top speed for a few seconds, then slower for recovery. At the high-gear level, the exercises should be performed mostly at top speed, though a warm-up and a tapering-off stage should always be included.

Usually, in any lesson, no muscular group is exercised to the point of exhaustion more than once in any five-minute period. First one muscular group is exercised, then another and another. In time, you may go back to exercising a muscular group that you exercised earlier, so that some repetitive work is done, usually at a higher level of effort. The principle is to work hard, ease off, work hard, ease off, and so on. This is "interval training" applied to ordinary exercising; it is the principle that makes continuity possible.

FREQUENCY OF WORKOUTS.   If you are in very poor condition, you may begin by taking one lesson per week, to learn form and style. But one lesson a week is not enough to insure any progress. Improvement of any appreciable amount demands that you work out a minimum of three times a week. Ideally, you should work out six times a week, and take the seventh day for some kind of lighter recreation like golf, bowling, dancing, or hiking.

SUPPLEMENTARY WORK.   The workouts may be supplemented by long walks, swims, bicycle rides, canoeing or rowing and any sports that you enjoy. However, to repeat, these activities should not be regarded as a substitute for the workouts. Various studies of professional athletes show that as soon as training ends and steady team competition begins, no further gains in fitness are achieved. Instead, there is a steady drain on the reserves. At the end of most playing seasons in basketball, football, baseball and other such sports, athletes are fatigued and in some cases have lower cardiovascular and respiratory fitness than they had at the beginning of the season.

You can also supplement the regular workout periods with special exercises designed to strengthen various parts of the body. A section of such exercises appears in the last chapter of this book.

AFTER YOU COMPLETE THE COURSE.   By the time you have completed the course, you will know enough about yourself, the various exercises and the amount of work you need to stay in shape to set up a permanent schedule of workouts. Three vigorous workouts a week are usually enough to keep you in top shape. The course will offer you sufficient variety so that you should have no trouble setting up a varied and interesting routine and deriving great satisfaction from your exercise.

Section I

A TWENTY–TWO–LESSON COURSE
OF PROGRESSIVE, RHYTHMICAL,
NON–STOP EXERCISES

1. The Twenty-two Lessons

LESSON 1. 30–MINUTE LOW–GEAR WORKOUT

The First Lesson is a typical low-gear exercise workout. It consists of a continuous (non-stop) conditioning workout that should last about thirty minutes. It is important that the exercises in this workout, and, in fact, all workouts, be performed without interruption. The exercises are always arranged so that this will be possible; slow, easy exercises are alternated with faster, more vigorous ones.

After a brief warm-up period, the plan is to work out the body progressively from top to bottom, beginning with the neck, arms and shoulders, and working down through the waist, lateral muscles, abdominal muscles, back muscles and the weight-bearing muscles of the feet and legs. This will be the general pattern throughout all of the lessons.

At first exercises demanding muscle tension will be generally avoided. You should concentrate on working at a slow, deliberate pace and consciously try to force your breathing, especially near the end of the lesson, when the exercises become slightly more vigorous. Breathing is most important; we will emphasize it again and again throughout the course.

I. WARM–UP EXERCISES (APPROXIMATELY 5 MINUTES)

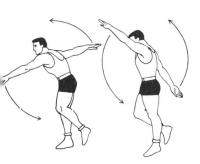

Walk and jog several laps around the gymnasium. Walk one lap, then jog one lap, then walk another lap and so on.

As you walk and jog, swing your arms in full circles, windmill fashion.

Also, force yourself to breathe deeply. Every so often, take a deep breath and hold it for a few seconds.

II. SHOULDER, ARM AND CHEST EXERCISES (APPROXIMATELY 8 MINUTES)

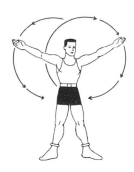

a. CROSS–BODY DOUBLE ARM CIRCLES   (1 MINUTE)

Starting position: Standing, with feet about one foot apart.

Movement: Swing arms upward and criss-cross in front of body in opposing circles as wide as possible. Shift weight from one foot to the other as you exercise.

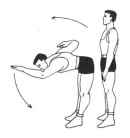

b. CRAWL STROKES, FORWARD   (1 MINUTE)

Starting position: Standing, feet slightly apart, bending forward from the waist.

Movement: Rotate arms in full forward alternate circles, much as if you were doing the crawl stroke.

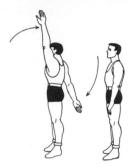

c. CRAWL STROKES, BACKWARD   (1 MINUTE)

Starting position: Standing upright, feet slightly apart.

Movement: Rotate arms in full backward alternate circles, as if you were doing the crawl stroke backward.

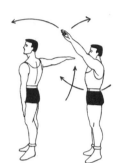

d. CJRCLING ONE ARM BACKWARD, THEN THE OTHER   (1 MINUTE)

Starting position: Standing upright.

Movement: Circle one arm backward about 10 times, then alternate. Repeat several times.

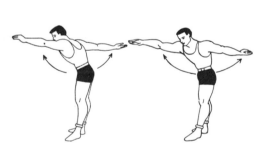

e. ARM SWINGING, FORWARD AND BACKWARD IN OPPOSITION   (1 MINUTE)

Starting position: Standing, bending forward from the waist with feet about 18 inches apart.

Movement: Simultaneously, swing right arm forward and left arm backward as far as they will go. Then reverse. Continue rhythmically, shifting weight from one foot to the other.

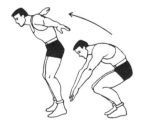

f. BUTTERFLY ARM STROKES   (1 MINUTE)

Starting position: Standing, feet together, bending forward from the waist.

Movement: Imitate the movements of the butterfly stroke in swimming: Pull both arms down and back, then circle them both forward in an overarm recovery. Go into a modified squat as you bring your arms down, and straighten up as you throw them up and out. Breathe as if you were actually in the water, taking an extra deep breath every third stroke.

g. SIMULTANEOUS ARM FLEXIONS   (1 MINUTE)

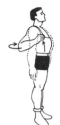

Starting position: Standing, feet about a foot apart, arms at sides.

Movement: With vigorous movements, flex both arms all the way, so that your hands are almost touching your armpits. Then swing your elbows back as far as they will go, so as to thrust your chest out. Bring your arms down to your side again. Repeat.

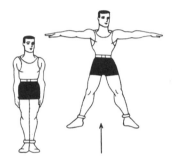

h. JUMPING JACKS   (1 MINUTE)

Starting position: Standing erect, with feet together, arms at your side.

Movement: In a single motion, jump off the ground and land with your feet about 2 feet apart; as you jump swing your arms up sideways and clap your hands together over your head. Then jump back to starting position. Repeat.

III. WAIST EXERCISES (APPROXIMATELY 4 MINUTES)

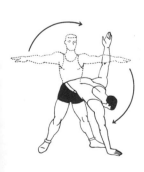

a. CROSS–BODY FLOOR TOUCHES   (2 MINUTES)

Starting position: Standing, with feet spread wide apart.

Movement: Swing your right arm overhead counterclockwise, then bend from the waist with knees stiff and touch your hand to the floor as far outside the left foot as possible. Then whip your arm back overhead, fast and hard, to original position, at the same time straightening up. Then repeat, using left arm to the opposite side. This should be one continuous movement. Exhale forcefully while touching the floor, and inhale while straightening up.

b. WAIST BENDS AND ROTATIONS   (2 MINUTES)

Starting position: Standing with feet apart, hands over head.

Movement: Bend down sharply and touch palms to floor 3 times, then swing both arms upward and to the left, making a sweeping, circular movement with the arms and the upper trunk, then return to starting position. Then repeat, swinging up in reverse direction. Continue, alternating directions.

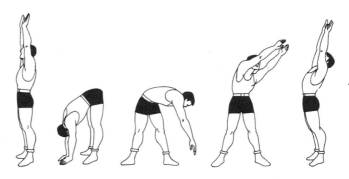

IV. ABDOMINAL, BACK AND LATERAL THIGH EXERCISES
(APPROXIMATELY 10 MINUTES)

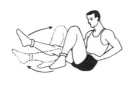

a. ALTERNATE KNEE–BEND KICKS   (1 MINUTE)

Starting position: Sitting, with legs extended and hands resting on floor next to hips.

Movement: Lift right leg slightly off the floor and bend until your heel is almost touching your right buttock. Then straighten your right leg, at the same time bending your left leg, almost as if you were bicycling. Keep repeating.

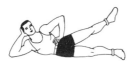

b. SIDE LEG KICKS   (1 MINUTE)

Starting position: Lying on the right side, with left hand on left hip and right hand supporting head.

Movement: Whip left leg up and down in rapid oscillating motion. At the top of the kick, your ankles should be about 15 inches apart. After kicking 25 to 30 times, turn over and repeat, using right leg.

c. FLUTTER KICKS   (2 MINUTES)

Starting position: Lying face down, with hands under thighs.

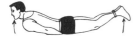

Movement: Raise your head and arch your back, then flutter-kick as if you were swimming, keeping your legs off the ground, your knees slightly bent, and your feet 10 to 15 inches apart. After about a minute of kicking, turn over on your back and repeat.

d. FORWARD BENDS, SITTING   (1 MINUTE)

Starting position: Sitting, with legs extended and hands clasped behind the neck.

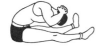

Movement: Bend forward as far as you can. Try to push your head out toward your feet and down. Then return to upright position and repeat.

e. TRUNK BENDS   (1 MINUTE)

Starting position: Standing, with feet about 18 inches apart, and with arms raised.

Movement: Bend forward and brush your fingertips to the floor. Do not force yourself beyond a comfortable point, even if it means that you don't touch the floor. Repeat.

f. SITTING TUCKS   (1 MINUTE)

Starting position: Sitting, with hands on floor beside hips and legs extended.

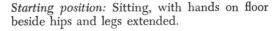

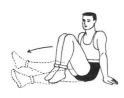

Movement: Draw both feet up simultaneously until your heels are almost touching your buttocks, and then thrust them out to extended position. Repeat.

g. CHEST LIFTS   (1 MINUTE)

Starting position: Lying on back, with hands on the floor beside hips.

Movement: Raise your chest, neck and head as far as possible from the floor and lower it again. Repeat.

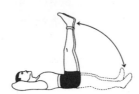

h. LEG LIFTS   (1 MINUTE)

Starting position: Lying on back with hands clasped behind neck.

Movement: Holding legs together, raise them to a vertical position, then lower slowly to the floor. Repeat.

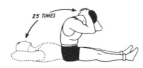

ı. SIT–UPS   (1 MINUTE)

Starting position: Lying on back, with hands clasped behind neck.

Movement: Sit up, and try to touch your shins with your elbows. Lie back. Repeat.

V. LEG AND FEET EXERCISES (APPROXIMATELY 5 MINUTES)

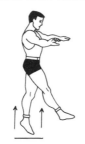

a. SKIP–KICKS IN PLACE—FORWARD   (1 MINUTE)

Starting position: Standing upright.

Movement: Skip in place (by hopping twice on one foot and then twice on the other). Instead of simply lifting your foot off the floor, kick it forward, keeping it relaxed.

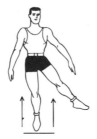

b. SKIP–KICKS IN PLACE—SIDEWAYS   (1 MINUTE)

Starting position: Standing upright.

Movement: Repeat above exercise, kicking sideways instead of forward.

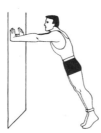

c. TOE PUSH–UPS   (1 MINUTE)

Starting position: Leaning with face toward wall, hands resting against wall chest high.

Movement: Stand up on tiptoes, then lower your heels to floor. Repeat 30 times.

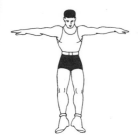

d. WALKING ON OUTSIDE OF FEET   (1 MINUTE)

Starting position: Standing on the outside edges of your feet.

Movement: Walk across gym or room floor, turn, walk back again.

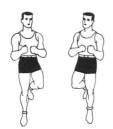

e. HOPPING ON ALTERNATE FEET   (1 MINUTE)

Starting position: Standing.

Movement: Hop for about 30 seconds on one foot, then hop for about 30 seconds on the other foot.

LESSON 2.   45-MINUTE LOW-GEAR WORKOUT

The Second Lesson introduces exercises which demand somewhat greater effort and a certain amount of tension. These more demanding exercises are preceded by a longer warm-up period, just as any strenuous exercise always should be. By the same token, the lesson ends with a five-minute tapering-off period, in which walking, deep breathing, stretching and balancing are stressed.

One valuable piece of advice: If an exercise (like arm circles or arm flexions) leaves you free to walk or jog while performing it, do so, for your system will circulate far more blood if you do. To illustrate: An adult performing an arm swinging exercise while standing uses about ten calories per hour per square meter of his body, while an adult performing the same exercise while running uses about three times as many calories.

Remember to exercise slowly and to breathe deeply and forcefully. This is still low gear.

I. WARM-UP EXERCISES (APPROXIMATELY 10 MINUTES)

a. CROSS-BODY DOUBLE ARM CIRCLES   (1 MINUTE)
See Lesson One, Exercise II a, page 103.

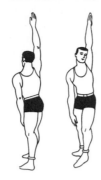

b. ARM STRETCHES WITH TRUNK TWISTS (1 MINUTE)

Starting position: Standing, with feet about a foot apart, arms at side.

Movement: Swing your right arm up to a vertical position beside or even somewhat behind your head, keeping your elbow straight. Then rotate your body a quarter turn to the right. Return to starting position. Then perform the same movement with your left arm. Repeat.

c. ARM SWINGING, FORWARD AND BACKWARD IN OPPOSITION   (1 MINUTE)

See Lesson One, Exercise II e, page 104.

d. CRAWL STROKES, FORWARD AND BACKWARD   (2 MINUTES)

See Lesson One, Exercises II b and II c, pages 103–04.

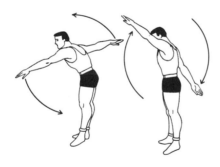

e. WINDMILLS, FORWARD AND BACKWARD   (1 MINUTE)

Starting position: Standing, bending forward from the waist, feet slightly apart.

Movement: Rotate arms forward, 180 degrees apart, in the anteroposterior plane. Begin slowly and speed up. Then reverse and perform the same exercise backward.

f. TRUNK BENDS   (1 MINUTE)

See Lesson One, Exercise IV e, page 107.

g. CROSS–BODY FLOOR TOUCHES   (1 MINUTE)

See Lesson One, Exercise III a, page 105.

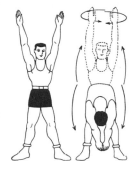

h. TRUNK FLEXIONS AND ROTATIONS   (1 MINUTE)

Starting position: Standing, with feet about 18 inches apart, arms extended overhead, and thumbs interlocked.

Movement: Bend forward from the waist and swing your arms down between your legs. Then straighten up and circle your hands on a horizontal plane above your head while rotating your upper trunk from the waist. Repeat, reversing the direction of the circles.

Now jog two laps around the gym, then walk one lap, all the while practicing deep breathing and stretching different parts of your body—flexing arms, kicking feet, and shaking hands overhead and at sides.

II. ABDOMINAL EXERCISES (APPROXIMATELY 10 MINUTES)

You will notice that four of the following exercises are accompanied by stretching exercises. The idea is to perform the exercise and then to stretch the muscles you have just finished exercising.

a. ALTERNATE KNEE–BEND KICKS AND STRETCH WITH TRUNK BENDS   (90 SECONDS)

For Alternate Knee-Bend Kicks, see Lesson One, Exercise IV a, page 106. For Trunk Bends, see Lesson One, Exercise IV e, page 107.

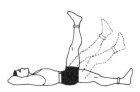

b. ALTERNATE SINGLE–LEG LIFTS AND BOW STRETCH   (90 SECONDS)

Starting position: Lying on back, with hands behind neck, legs extended straight.

Movement: Raise your right leg to a vertical position, then lower it slowly. Then do the same thing with your left leg. Repeat for one minute. Then roll over onto your stomach, put your hands behind your neck, and arch your body, raising your chest and legs as far off the floor as you can.

c. SITTING TUCKS AND STRETCH BY SIT SPRINGING   (90 SECONDS)

For Sitting Tucks, see Lesson One, Exercise IV f, page 107.

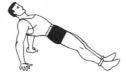

The stretch is performed by getting into a sitting position, with the hands on floor about 12 inches behind you, then raising your trunk as far as you can, so that your weight is supported on your hands and heels. Flex your back a few times while breathing deeply.

d. LEG LIFTS AND STRETCH WITH FORWARD BENDS, SITTING   (90 SECONDS)

For Leg Lifts, see Lesson One, Exercise IV h, page 108.
For Forward Bends Sitting, see Lesson One, Exercise IV d, page 107. (Occasionally, place an 8-inch-high book between your knees, and try to touch your forehead to the book.)

e. SIT–UPS WITH HANDS AT SIDES   (1 MINUTE)

Starting position: Lying on back, with hands at sides.

Movement: Sit up, stretch forward, and lower your head as far as possible; return to prone position. Repeat.

f. Now walk and skip-kick one lap around the gym, then walk one lap, all the while practicing deep breathing and stretching different parts of your body.

III. ARM AND SHOULDER EXERCISES (APPROXIMATELY 16 MINUTES)

Some of the following exercises require special equipment usually found in well-equipped gyms. One exercise requires a partner. Obviously, if you are working out at home, you will have to skip these exercises. In some cases, you will find that you can substitute another exercise which taxes the same muscles.

a. KNEE PUSH–UPS   (1 MINUTE)

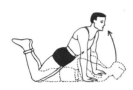

Starting position: Lying on floor, face down, with legs together, knees bent 90 degrees, and hands on floor under shoulders, palms down.

Movement: Push the upper part of your body off the floor until your arms are fully extended. At this point, your body should be a straight line from your knees to your head. Then lower yourself until chin or chest touches floor. Repeat continuously.
(This exercise is preparation for full push-ups.)

b. PULLEY WEIGHTS   (5 MINUTES)

Work out with pulley weights for about five minutes. There are a number of different exercises to build up strength in the arms and shoulders. (See Special Exercises: Part Two, Chapter 6, Section VI —pages 176–77.)

c. CRAWL STROKES, FORWARD   (1 MINUTE)

See Lesson One, Exercise II b, page 103.

d. ROWING MACHINE   (5 MINUTES)

Work out on a rowing machine for about five minutes.

e. BAR HANG   (1 MINUTE)

Simply grasp a horizontal bar with both hands and hang freely (with feet off the floor) for one minute. (This is a preparatory exercise for chin-ups.)

f. FOREARM PRESS–UPS   (1 MINUTE)

Starting position: Lying face down, with arms fully extended, forearms on the floor.

Movement: Keeping your body straight, press yourself up as far as you can, until you are resting on your toes and forearms. Then return to starting position. Repeat continuously.

g. WHEELBARROW WALK
(WITH PARTNER)   (2 MINUTES)

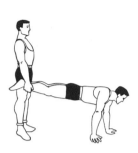

Starting position: Front leaning rest, with partner standing and grasping your ankles as he would the handles of a wheelbarrow.

Movement: Walk on your hands the width of the gymnasium. Then reverse positions and walk back.
h. Now jog one lap around the gym, then walk one lap, all the while breathing deeply and stretching different parts of your body. (In a small room jog in place.)

IV. LEG AND FEET EXERCISES (APPROXIMATELY 6 MINUTES)

a. LEANING STRETCH   (1 MINUTE)

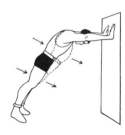

Starting position: Leaning with face toward wall, hands resting on wall higher than head-level, and feet at least three feet from wall.

Movement: Keeping your arms straight, and your feet in place, press your torso toward the wall as far as you can. Then return to starting position and repeat.

b. TOE PUSH-UPS   (1 MINUTE)

See Lesson One, Exercise V c, page 108.

c. QUARTER KNEE BENDS   (1 MINUTE)

Starting position: Standing.

Movement: Go into a modified squatting position with your knees bent about 45 degrees. Return to starting position. Repeat continuously.

d. WALKING ON OUTSIDES OF FEET   (1 MINUTE)

See Lesson One, Exercise V d, page 109.

e. HOPPING ON ALTERNATE FEET **(1 MINUTE)**

See Lesson One, Exercise V e, page 109.

f. VERTICAL JUMPS **(1 MINUTE)**

Starting position: Standing.

Movement: Swing your arms downward and crouch down; then spring up as high as you can. With one hand try to hit an imaginary spot on the wall. Repeat.

V. TAPERING–OFF EXERCISE (APPROXIMATELY 5 MINUTES)

Jog one lap around gym, then walk five laps while practicing deep breathing and stretching the different parts of your body. At one point in each lap, raise one arm and hold your breath for 15 paces. Then inhale and exhale forcefully for about a minute.

LESSON 3. 30–MINUTE LOW–GEAR WORKOUT

As we pointed out in the introduction to these lessons, this fitness course progresses from low gear to middle gear to high gear. As we also pointed out, the rate of progression from one lesson to the next will depend on the physical condition of the class. By this point in the program you will have begun to notice that each lesson requires a little more exertion than the one preceding it. The idea is, of course, to make the build-up as gradual as possible, so that the person taking the course can adapt himself without strain.

You will also have noticed by now that the exercises within each lesson progress from low to middle to high gear. This is to warm up the circulatory and respiratory systems before undertaking any high-tension exercises. Even professional athletes do this.

At some point in each lesson, we introduce a few exercises that appear later, at a more intense level, in order to give you a taste of what they're like. The harder exercises should only be tried for a few seconds, especially at the early stages, for if you strain yourself for more than a brief period the consequences can be serious.

Actually, you will be kept away from high-tension exercises for a month or two. At this stage, continue to concentrate on correct breathing until it comes naturally.

I. WARM–UP EXERCISES (APPROXIMATELY 10 MINUTES)

a. WALK AND JOG AROUND THE GYM   (5 MINUTES)

See.Lesson One, Exercise I, page 103.

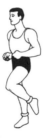

b. RUNNING IN PLACE   (5 MINUTES)

Starting position: Standing.

Movement: Run in place as vigorously as you can, lifting your feet at least 5 inches off the floor. While you are running breathe forcefully and deeply. Start slowly and speed up a little at one minute intervals.

II. SHOULDER, ARM AND CHEST EXERCISES (APPROXIMATELY 8 MINUTES)

a. CROSS–BODY DOUBLE ARM CIRCLES   (1 MINUTE)

See Lesson One, Exercise II a, page 103.

b. CRAWL STROKES, FORWARD   (1 MINUTE)

See Lesson One, Exercise II b, page 103.

c. CRAWL STROKES, BACKWARD   (1 MINUTE)

See Lesson One, Exercise II c, page 104.

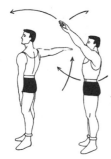

d. LARGE ARM-CIRCLES (1 MINUTE)

Starting position: Standing, with arms at sides.

Movement: Rotate your right arm in full circles in an anteroposterior plane, somewhat as if you were winding up to pitch a softball. Repeat in the opposite direction. Then do the same thing with the other arm.

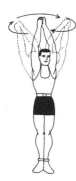

e. SMALL ARM-CIRCLES (1 MINUTE)

Starting position: Standing, with arms extended over head and hands clasped.

Movement: Rotate arms rapidly in small circles over your head. Make 10 circles to the right, then 10 circles to the left. Repeat.

f. KNEE PUSH-UPS (1 MINUTE)

See Lesson Two, Exercise III a, page 113.

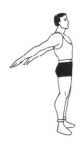

g. ARM EXTENSION, BACKWARD (1 MINUTE)

Starting position: Standing with arms at sides.

Movement: Pull your arms backward as far as they will go without bending your head or shoulders. Hold this position as long as you can.

h. JUMPING JACKS (1 MINUTE)

See Lesson One, Exercise II h, page 105.

III. WAIST EXERCISES (APPROXIMATELY 3 MINUTES)

a. CROSS-BODY FLOOR TOUCHES (1 MINUTE)

See Lesson One, Exercise III a, page 105.

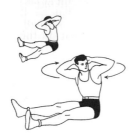

b. TORSO ROTATION, SITTING   **(1 MINUTE)**

Starting position: Sitting on floor, with legs extended to the front and arms extended to the sides.

Movement: Twist the upper part of your body to the left as far as you can, then rotate to the right. Repeat.

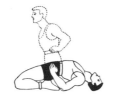

c. BACK FLEXIONS   **(1 MINUTE)**

Starting position: Kneeling, with buttocks back on heels and with hands on hips.

Movement: Lean back as far as you can and flex your back by arching backward. Repeat.

IV. ABDOMINAL, LOWER BACK AND WAIST EXERCISES (APPROXIMATELY 8 MINUTES)

a. SIDE LEG–KICKS   **(2 MINUTES)**

See Lesson One, Exercise IV b, page 106.

b. FLUTTER KICKS   **(1 MINUTE)**

See Lesson One, Exercise IV c, page 107.

c. TRUNK BENDS   **(1 MINUTE)**

See Lesson One, Exercise IV e, page 107.

d. SITTING TUCKS   **(1 MINUTE)**

See Lesson One, Exercise IV f, page 107.

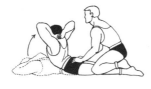

**e. CHEST LIFTS (WITH PARTNER,
IF AVAILABLE)**   **(2 MINUTES)**

Starting position: Lying face down, with hands behind neck, partner kneeling across legs to hold them down.

Movement: Raise your chest, neck and head as far as possible from the floor and lower it again. Repeat.

f. SIT–UPS   **(1 MINUTE)**

See Lesson One, Exercise IV i, page 108.

V. TAPERING–OFF EXERCISES (APPROXIMATELY 5 MINUTES)

Jog one lap around gym, then walk five laps while practicing deep breathing and stretching different parts of your body. At one point in each lap, raise one arm and hold your breath for 20 paces. Then inhale and exhale forcefully for about a minute.

LESSON 4. 40–MINUTE LOW-GEAR WORKOUT

The Fourth Lesson concentrates on two exercises which are designed to build up endurance. The basic plan of the workout is arranged to have you exercise for one minute; then stop for one minute to rest, breathe deeply and stretch; exercise for two minutes; stop for one minute to rest, breathe and stretch; exercise for three minutes; and rest, breathe and stretch. Actually, it's a little more complicated than that, but if you follow the program or your instructor, you won't have any problem. The important thing is to build up your effort gradually in order to avoid muscle strain.

If possible, you should measure your pulse rate and your blood pressure before and after this workout. A comparison of the two sets of readings will indicate the degree of stress built up and the amount of adjustment to prolonged exercise you have made.

I. WARM–UP EXERCISE (APPROXIMATELY 10 MINUTES)

a. Walk with long strides on a treadmill. It should be adjusted to an 8.6 per cent grade and a speed of 3 to 4 mph.

b. Rest, breathe deeply, and perform a stretching exercise for one minute.

II. ENDURANCE EXERCISES (APPROXIMATELY 24 MINUTES)

a. Row on a push-pull type rowing machine for *one minute*. (You should row at the rate of 30 strokes per minute.)
Rest, breathe and stretch for *one minute*.

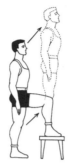

b. BENCH STEPPING

Starting position: Standing, in front of a chair or bench approximately 14 inches high.

Movement: Place your right foot on the bench, bring your left foot onto bench and stand up, lower your right foot to the floor, and then lower your left foot to the floor. Repeat continuously for *one minute*. Then reverse feet and repeat.

Rest, breathe and stretch for *one minute*.

c. Repeat exercise on rowing machine for *two minutes*.
Rest, breathe and stretch for *one minute*.

d. Repeat bench-stepping exercise for *two minutes*.
Rest, breathe and stretch for *one minute*.

e. Repeat exercise on rowing machine for *two minutes*.
Rest, breathe and stretch for *one minute*.

f. Repeat bench-stepping exercise for *three minutes*.
Rest, breathe and stretch for *one minute*.

g. Repeat exercise on rowing machine for *three minutes*.
Rest, breathe and stretch for *one minute*.

h. Repeat bench-stepping exercise for *three minutes*.
Rest, breathe and stretch for *one minute*.

III. TAPERING–OFF EXERCISES (APPROXIMATELY 5 MINUTES)

See Lesson Three, Exercise V a, page 119.

LESSON 5.   60–MINUTE LOW–GEAR WORKOUT

The Fifth Lesson extends the length of the workouts from forty minutes to a full hour, and includes exercises requiring both special equipment and partners.

This is as good a point as any to review briefly some of the practical points about cardiovascular fitness. You are probably aware of how essential a part of physical fitness cardiovascular fitness is. Good cardiovascular condition can be developed by long-drawn-out endurance exercises gradually approached by longer and longer drill sessions. A sound training program will bring about improvements in a number of components of cardiovascular fitness. These include a strong heart stroke, a larger flow of blood through the central circulatory system, a lower pulse rate, a greater ability to adjust to changes of position, a greater capacity to recover from intense expenditure of energy and the capacity to expend more energy.

As the lessons proceed, you will begin to notice the appearance of exercises specifically designed to improve your cardiovascular system.

I. WARM–UP EXERCISES (APPROXIMATELY 20 MINUTES)

a. Walk one lap around gym, then jog one lap.
   Walk one lap, then jog two laps.
   Walk one lap, then jog three laps.
   Walk one lap, then jog four laps.
   Walk one lap, then jog five laps.

b. Walk two laps while practicing deep breathing and stretching different parts of your body.

II. BODY EXERCISES (APPROXIMATELY 15 MINUTES)

The following five exercises require you to work with a partner. If you are working with a large formal class, the instructor should line the group up and have it count off: "One," "two," "one," "two," and so on down the line. Each "one" should then pair off with a "two," who will act as his partner.

If you are working out on your own, you can perform the exercises by yourself. In this case, the group of exercises should take about half the time allotted.

a. CHEST LIFTS (WITH PARTNER)   (2 MINUTES)

See Lesson Three, Exercise IV e, page 118.
Perform the exercise 15 times and then switch positions.

b. SIT–UPS (WITH PARTNER)   (2 MINUTES)

See Lesson One, Exercise IV i, page 108.
Your partner should sit on your legs. Perform 15 times and then switch
positions.

c. ALTERNATE SINGLE–LEG LIFTS (WITH PARTNER)   (2 MINUTES)

See Lesson Two, Exercise II b, page 111 (without Bow Stretch).
Your partner should kneel at your head and pin down your elbows.
Perform 15 times and then switch positions.

d. LEG LIFTS (WITH PARTNER)   (2 MINUTES)

See Lesson One, Exercise IV h, page 108.
Your partner should pin down your elbows. Perform 15 times and then
switch positions.

e. TRUNK LIFTS SIDEWAYS (WITH PARTNER)   (4 MINUTES)

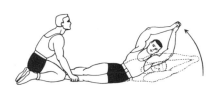

Starting position: Lying on left side, with arms extended above head and partner pinning down legs.

Movement: Raise the upper part of your body as far off the floor as you can. Do this 15 times on each side, then switch positions with your partner.

III. FOOT AND LEG EXERCISES (APPROXIMATELY 5 MINUTES)

a. WALKING ON OUTSIDE OF FEET   (1 MINUTE)

See Lesson One, Exercise V d, page 109.

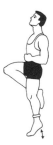

b. TOE–HEEL PRANCE

Starting position: Standing.

Movement: Run forward, bringing your knees up as high as you can, landing on the balls of your feet, and lowering the heel of your foot to the ground before each succeeding step. Do one lap.

c. Hop the length of the gym on the right foot only. (1 minute)

d. Hop the length of the gym on the left foot only. (1 minute)

IV. POSTURE EXERCISES (APPROXIMATELY 5 MINUTES)

a. BACK STRAIGHTENER   (1 MINUTE)

Starting position: Lying flat on back, with arms at sides.

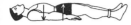

Movement: Take a deep breath, and flatten the lower part of your back to the floor for five seconds, then relax. Repeat 10 times, exhaling fully with release.

b. TOE PUSH–UPS   (1 MINUTE)

See Lesson One, Exercise V c, page 108.

c. SIDE LEG–KICKS, HIGHER   (1 MINUTE ON EACH SIDE)

See Lesson One, Exercise IV b, page 106, but kick upper leg as high as you can.

d. SITTING TUCKS   (1 MINUTE)

See Lesson One, Exercise IV f, page 107.

V. HAND AND SHOULDER EXERCISES (APPROXIMATELY 10 MINUTES)

Three of the following exercises require the use of a vertical ladder-like fixture called a stall bar, which you will find in most gymnasiums.

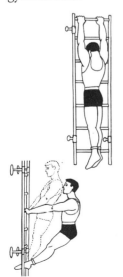

a. With hands grasping the top stall bar, hang with your feet off the ground for one minute.

b. FULL HAMSTRING STRETCH   (1 MINUTE)

Starting position: Standing on lowest stall bar, facing bars, with legs straight and with hands grasping vertical bars about waist high.

Movement: Keeping your legs straight, swing back and down as far as you can. Then pull yourself back to starting position, and repeat.

c. UPSIDE–DOWN BICYCLE   (1 MINUTE)

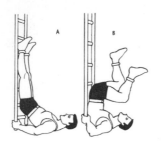

Starting position: Resting on shoulders, with legs extended and propped up against the stall bar, and with hands grasping bases of vertical bars.

Movement: Pull yourself up against stall bar so that your lower back rests against bars, your shoulders and upper arms are resting on the floor, and your legs are free. Then move your legs as if you were peddling a bicycle.

d. Work out on rowing machine (5 minutes)
> or

work out with pulley weights
> or

do Knee Push-Ups (See Lesson Two, Exercise III a, page 113).
> or

throw *medicine ball* (with partner or against a wall) (See Special Exercises: Part Two, Chapter 6, Section V—page 175).

VI. TAPERING–OFF EXERCISE (APPROXIMATELY 5 MINUTES)

Run on treadmill or on floor, gradually slowing down to a walk and then a standstill. Then assume a diver's stance—on tiptoes, with heels together, arms extended in front of you, and eyes closed—and hold for 20 seconds.

LESSON 6. 60–MINUTE LOW–GEAR WORKOUT

The Sixth Lesson introduces special exercises in breathing and breath holding. Breathing is emphasized here and throughout the various lessons because in order to achieve physical fitness you must develop the habit of breathing regularly while exercising so that you will (1) avoid fatigue, and (2) increase the capacity of your respiratory system.

If you pay close attention to yourself while you exercise you will find that you have a natural tendency to hold your breath, particularly when you are performing high-tension or unfamiliar exercises. Rather than capturing more air in your lungs and thereby giving you greater endurance, holding your breath only serves to deplete the supply of oxygen, speed up the accumulation of carbon dioxide, and cause your muscles to become fatigued more quickly. The habit of breathing regularly during all forms of exercise can be developed through conscious practice of deep inhalation and forced exhalation.

Breathing drills also help to build up lung capacity. A deep breath held for a few seconds will increase the air pressure in the lungs by forcing air into lung tissue that is not normally active in breathing. And the drills that are introduced in this lesson will help your lung capacity by getting you to breathe regularly and fully during all forms of exertion.

I. WARM–UP EXERCISES (APPROXIMATELY 20 MINUTES)

a. Walk one lap around gym, then jog one lap.
    Walk one lap, then jog two laps.
    Walk one lap, then jog four laps.
    Walk one lap, then jog six laps.
    Walk one lap, then jog eight laps.
b. Now walk two laps around gym, all the while breathing deeply and stretching your arms, chest, and shoulders.

II. STRETCHING EXERCISES (APPROXIMATELY 6 MINUTES)

The following exercises require you to work with a partner. If you are working with a large formal class, the instructor should divide you up into pairs (See Lesson Five, Exercise II, pages 121–22).

a. FACE–TO–FACE STRETCH   (2 MINUTES)

Starting position: Sitting, facing your partner and grasping his hands, with legs extended so that your feet are against his feet.

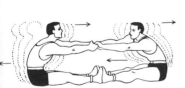

Movement: Pull your partner's hands as hard as you can, while he bends his trunk toward you. Then bend your trunk toward your partner as he pulls you.

b. FEET–TO–FEET STRETCH   (2 MINUTES)

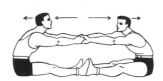

Starting position: Sitting, facing your partner and grasping his hands, with legs extended so that your feet are against his feet.

Movement: Pull your partner's arms as hard as you can, while he pulls against you.

c. BACK–TO–BACK STRETCH   (2 MINUTES)

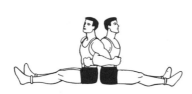
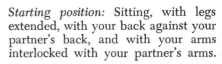

Starting position: Sitting, with legs extended, with your back against your partner's back, and with your arms interlocked with your partner's arms.

Movement: Pull your partner's arms as hard as you can, while he pulls against you.

III. BREATHING AND BREATH–HOLDING EXERCISES (APPROXIMATELY 6 MINUTES)

a. Run in place for 2 minutes, then sit down and hold your breath 10 seconds. Do this by taking 3 deep breaths and holding the third breath. Mark the seconds by slapping your hand on your thigh.

b. BACK STRAIGHTENER—HOLDING BREATH   (1 MINUTE)

Starting position: Lying flat on back, with arms at sides.

Movement: Take a deep breath, hold it, and flatten the lower part of your back to the floor for 5 seconds. Repeat 10 times, exhaling fully with release. Then bend one leg, grasp knee with both hands, and pull. Repeat with your other leg.

c. Run in place for 2 minutes, then hold your breath 15 seconds.

d. BACK STRAIGHTENER—HOLDING BREATH   (1 MINUTE)

Repeat Exercise III b.

IV. HARD BODY EXERCISES (APPROXIMATELY 10 MINUTES)

a. SITTING TUCKS   **(30 TIMES; 1 MINUTE)**

See Lesson One, Exercise IV f, page 107.

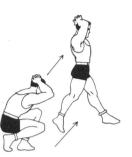

b. SQUAT JUMPS   **(30 TIMES; 1 MINUTE)**

Starting position: Standing, with one foot forward and one foot back and hands resting on top of head with fingers interlaced.

Movement: Lower yourself into a full squat, keeping your back straight and vertical. Then straighten yourself with enough thrust so that you jump off the ground. At the top of your jump shift the forward foot back and the backward foot forward. Repeat.

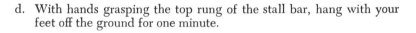

c. SIDE LEANING LEG LIFTS   **(2 MINUTES)**

Starting position: Leaning on one side, with body supported by straight arm and side of lower foot.

Movement: Raise upper leg until it is parallel to floor and lower. Repeat. Turn over and do the same thing on other side.

d. With hands grasping the top rung of the stall bar, hang with your feet off the ground for one minute.

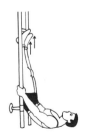

e. STALL–BAR LEG PRESS   **(1 MINUTE)**

Starting position: Resting on shoulders, with legs extended up stall bar, feet pressed on bottom of bar, and hands grasping bases of vertical bars.

Movement: Press your feet against the bar and your shoulders against the floor, and count to three. Release pressure for count of three and reapply pressure. Repeat 15 times.

f. Work on rowing machine, pulley weights, push-ups, or medicine ball (See Special Exercises: Part Two, Chapter 6, Section V—pages 172–77.)

VI. TAPERING–OFF EXERCISE (APPROXIMATELY 5 MINUTES)

Run on treadmill or on floor, gradually slowing down to a walk and then a standstill. Then perform a three-point headstand for 30 seconds.

LESSON 7. 60–MINUTE LOW–GEAR WORKOUT

A large part of Lesson Seven is devoted to what we refer to as hard body exercises. As you will note, some of these exercises have already appeared in previous lessons. They will appear more and more throughout the remaining lessons.

The purpose of hard exercising is to increase strength. In order to increase the strength of a muscle it must be *repeatedly exerted more than half of its maximum capacity*. Even a great deal of low-level effort will not develop strength. The two most important ways of achieving the necessary exertion of a muscle are (1) exercising it with *speed* and (2) exercising it with *resistance*. Thus, the hard body exercises that we recommend emphasize increasing speed as the lessons progress, and involve methods of applying the necessary resistance.

The arms may be strengthened by lifting your own body weight (on a chinning bar, on the stall bar, or by climbing a rope), by working with pulley weights, a rowing machine, a medicine ball, or bar bells. The legs may be strengthened by stepping onto and off of a chair, by running uphill, by half squats or toe raises. The abdominal muscles may be strengthened by pulling them forcefully inward, by forcing the abdomen outward against some resistance (with glottis closed), by rapid leg lifts and sit-ups. The lateral muscles may be developed by rapid side leg-kicks, by sideway trunk lifts, by putting the shot or a medicine ball for distance. The hip and thigh flexor muscles may be strengthened by running, hopping and squat jumping. All of these exercises involve some resistance either in the form of your own body or some object.

As a general rule, the harder the exercise, the greater the development of strength; the longer the exercise, the greater the development of cardiovascular efficiency—*provided the exercise is within the individual's range of ability.*

I. WARM–UP EXERCISES (APPROXIMATELY 20 MINUTES)

a. Walk one fast lap, then jog two laps.
    Walk one fast lap, then jog three laps.
    Walk one fast lap, then jog four laps.
    Walk one fast lap, then jog five laps.
b. Now walk two laps around gym, all the while breathing deeply and stretching your arms, chest and shoulders with pumping, shaking and stretching movements.

II. STRETCHING EXERCISES (APPROXIMATELY 6 MINUTES)

The following exercises require you to work with a partner. If you are working with a large formal class, the instructor should divide you into pairs (See Lesson Five, Exercises II, pages 121–22).

a. FACE–TO–FACE STRETCH   **(2 MINUTES)**

See Lesson Six, Exercise II a, page 125.

b. FEET–TO–FEET STRETCH   **(2 MINUTES)**

See Lesson Six, Exercise II b, page 126.

c. BACK–TO–BACK STRETCH   **(2 MINUTES)**

See Lesson Six, Exercise II c, page 126.

III. BREATHING AND BREATH–HOLDING EXERCISES (APPROXI-MATELY 6 MINUTES)

a. Sitting down, take 3 deep breaths and hold third breath for 15 seconds. Repeat for 20 seconds.
b. Jog two laps around gym, sit down, take 3 deep breaths and hold third breath for 30 seconds.

c. BACK STRAIGHTENER—HOLDING BREATH (1 MINUTE)

See Lesson Six, Exercise III b, page 126.

IV. HARD BODY EXERCISES (APPROXIMATELY 30 MINUTES)

Again, some of the following exercises require you to work with a partner.

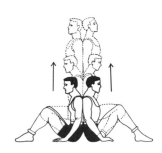

a. BACK–TO–BACK PRESS AND STAND (WITH PARTNER) (2 MINUTES)

Starting position: Sitting, with knees bent enough to allow feet to get traction on floor and with back to partner in same position.

Movement: Push yourself against your partner's back until you have reached a standing position. Perform this movement with maximum resistance, so that it takes about 2 minutes to reach a standing position.

b. MEDICINE BALL EXERCISES (12 MINUTES)

Starting position: Standing, facing your partner. (If you are working in a large class, your instructor should have the class form two lines facing each other.)

Movement: Throw a medicine ball to your partner, and catch it when he throws it back. Spend 3 minutes throwing it with a two-handed overhead throw, 3 minutes with a one-handed underhand throw, 3 minutes with a two-handed chest pass, and 3 minutes shot-putting it.

c. FLUTTER KICKS (2 MINUTES)

See Lesson One, Exercise IV c, page 107.

d. LEG SPREAD (2 MINUTES)

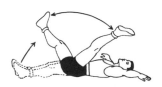

Starting position: Lying on back, with arms at sides and legs extended together straight and lifted far enough off the floor to form a 45-degree angle.

Movement: Keeping your legs in the air, spread them as far apart as is comfortable, then bring them together again, then lower to floor. Repeat until you are tired.

e. SIT–UPS   **(2 MINUTES)**

See Lesson One, IV i, page 108.

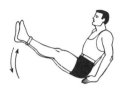

f. V–SITS   **(1 MINUTE)**

Starting position: Sitting on floor, with legs extended together and with hands on floor beside hips.

Movement: Keeping both legs and torso straight, lift legs and upper body off the floor until your body forms a modified V. Hold for one minute.

g. CIRCULAR STRETCH   **(1 MINUTE)**

Starting position: Lying on stomach, with hands grasping ankles behind back.

Movement: Push and pull against your ankles as hard as you can for one minute.

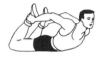

h. STOMACH ROCK   **(1 MINUTE)**

Starting position: Same as preceding exercise.

Movement: Rock forward and backward for one minute.

i. UPSIDE–DOWN BICYCLE (WITHOUT STALL BAR)   **(1 MINUTE)**

See Lesson Five, Exercise V c, page 124. Instead of propping yourself up against stall bar, prop yourself up with your hands on your waist and your elbows on the floor.

j. TORSO ROTATION, SITTING   **(1 MINUTE)**

See Lesson Three, Exercise III b, page 118. On each rotation to the right and left, add a little extra twist before rotating in the opposite direction.

V. TAPERING–OFF EXERCISES (APPROXIMATELY 5 MINUTES)

Run on treadmill or on floor, gradually slowing down to a walk and then a standstill. Then perform a handstand, with heels propped against the wall, for 30 seconds.

LESSON 8. 60–MINUTE MIDDLE–GEAR WORKOUT

The Eighth Lesson marks the beginning of the transition from low-gear exercising to middle-gear exercising. Up to this point you should have been performing the various exercises in a slow and measured manner, concentrating more on regular breathing than on speed. The transition to middle gear is made by approximately doubling the speed of the movements made in the exercises. This change of rate should be accomplished by beginning each individual exercise at a slow pace and midway through it (at a signal from the instructor if you are working in a class), doubling the rate of speed for a short time. This period of increased speed should last longer and longer as the workouts progress. This schedule fits into the routine well because the intervals of slower exercising may be used as warming-up and tapering-off periods. Gradual tapering-off is particularly important in the continuous, non-stop variety of workout which is featured in the entire series of lessons.

I. WARM–UP EXERCISES (APPROXIMATELY 10 MINUTES)

Walk one lap around gym, then run two laps, breathing forcefully.
Walk one lap, then run four laps, breathing forcefully.
Walk one lap, then run six laps, breathing forcefully.
Walk one lap, then run eight laps, breathing forcefully.
Walk one lap, then run ten laps, breathing forcefully.
Walk three laps, breathing forcefully.

II. SHOULDER, ARM AND CHEST EXERCISES (APPROXIMATELY 10 MINUTES)

See Lesson One, Section II, page 103. Each exercise should be started at slow pace, then accelerated for longer and longer periods.

III. WAIST EXERCISES (APPROXIMATELY 5 MINUTES)

See Lesson One, Section III, pages 105–06. Apply speed transition as above.

IV. ABDOMINAL, BACK AND LATERAL THIGH EXERCISES (APPROXIMATELY 10 MINUTES)

See Lesson One, Section IV, pages 106–08. Apply speed transition.

V. LEG AND FEET EXERCISES (APPROXIMATELY 10 MINUTES)

See Lesson One, Section V, pages 108–09. Apply speed transition.

VI. ARM EXERCISES (APPROXIMATELY 10 MINUTES)

See Lesson Five, Exercise V d, page 124.

VII. TAPERING–OFF AND RECOVERY EXERCISES (APPROXIMATELY 5 MINUTES)

At will, walk, shower and rest.

LESSON 9. 60–MINUTE MIDDLE–GEAR WORKOUT

Lesson Nine should complete the transition to middle-gear exercising. By the time that you have completed the previous lesson and gotten well into this lesson, the middle-gear rate should be predominant during the major part of the workout—about twice the speed at which you were exercising at the start of the course.

I. WARM–UP EXERCISES (APPROXIMATELY 15 MINUTES)

Walk one lap around gym, then run two laps.
Walk one lap, then run four laps.
Walk one lap, then run six laps.
Walk one lap, then run eight laps.
Walk one lap, then run ten laps.
Walk one lap, then jog two leisurely laps breathing deeply and stretching.

II. SHOULDER, ARM AND CHEST EXERCISES (APPROXIMATELY 6 MINUTES)

a. CIRCLING ONE ARM BACKWARD, THEN THE OTHER　　　(1 MINUTE)

See Lesson One, Exercise II d, page 104.

b. LARGE ARM–CIRCLES AND SMALL ARM–CIRCLES　　　(2 MINUTES)

For Large Arm-Circles, see Lesson Three, Exercise II d, page 117.
For Small Arm-Circles, see Lesson Three, Exercise II e, page 117.

c. CRAWL STROKES, FORWARD　　　(1 MINUTE)

See Lesson One, Exercise II b, page 103.

d. CRAWL STROKES, BACKWARD　　　(1 MINUTE)

See Lesson One, Exercise II c, page 104.

e. CROSS–BODY DOUBLE ARM CIRCLES　　　(1 MINUTE)

See Lesson One, Exercise II a, page 103.

f. Now jog two laps, all the while breathing deeply and stretching your arms, chest and shoulders. Then go to a chinning bar and chin yourself almost to the limit of your ability.

III. WAIST AND HIP EXERCISES (APPROXIMATELY 10 MINUTES)

a. SIT–UPS　　　(1 MINUTE)

See Lesson One, Exercise IV i, page 108. (Do 60)

b. TORSO ROTATION, SITTING　　　(2 MINUTES)

See Lesson Three, Exercise III b, page 118. (Do 30 each way).

c. V–SITS　　　(1 MINUTE)

See Lesson Seven, Exercise IV f, page 131.

d. CHEST LIFTS (WITH PARTNER)   **(1 MINUTE)**

See Lesson Three, Exercise IV e, page 118.

e. TRUNK LIFTS SIDEWAYS (WITH PARTNER)   **(2 MINUTES)**

See Lesson Five, Exercise II e, page 122.

f. Run two laps around gym. At the start of each lap, hold your breath for thirty paces, exhale sharply, and breathe forcefully.

IV. ABDOMEN, BACK AND LATERAL TRUNK EXERCISES (APPROXIMATELY 10 MINUTES)

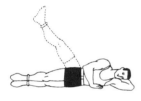

a. ALTERNATE-SIDE LEG LIFTS   **(2 MINUTES)**

Starting position: Lying on left side, with legs extended, left hand supporting head.

Movement: Whip your right leg up as far as it will go and lower again. Repeat, then reverse sides.

b. SITTING TUCKS   **(1 MINUTE)**

See Lesson One, Exercise IV f, page 107.

c. LEG LIFTS   **(2 MINUTES)**

See Lesson One, Exercise IV h, page 108.

d. LEG SPREAD   **(1 MINUTE)**

See Lesson Seven, Exercise IV d, page 130.

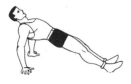

e. BACK HIP RAISES   **(1 MINUTE)**

Starting position: Back toward floor, with heels and hands supporting body.

Movement: Whip midsection up and down in rapid movement.

f. Run three laps around gym. Then walk one lap, hold breath for thirty paces, exhale sharply, and breathe forcefully for one minute.

V. FEET AND LEG EXERCISES (APPROXIMATELY 8 MINUTES)

a. Skip one lap around gym.

b. With feet together jump one lap around gym.

c. WALKING ON OUTSIDE OF FEET   (1 MINUTE)

See Lesson One, Exercise V d, page 109.

d. TOE PUSH–UPS   (1 MINUTE)

See Lesson One, Exercise V c, page 108.

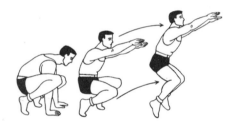

e. PROGRESSIVE LEAPS   (1 MINUTE)

Starting position: Full squat, hands on floor.

Movement: Throw both arms forward and up, and leap as far forward as you can. Repeat 10 times.

f. VERTICAL JUMPS   (2 MINUTES)

See Lesson Two, Exercise IV f, page 115.

g. Run two laps around gym. Then walk one lap, breathing forcefully and shaking out your limbs.

VI. ARM EXERCISES (APPROXIMATELY 10 MINUTES)

MEDICINE BALL EXERCISES   (10 MINUTES)

See Lesson Seven, Exercise IV b, page 130.

VII. TAPERING–OFF EXERCISES (APPROXIMATELY 5 MINUTES)

Walk, breathe deeply, take a cold shower and relax enough to rest and refresh yourself.

LESSON 10. 60–MINUTE MIDDLE–GEAR WORKOUT

Lesson Ten demonstrates the technique of circuit training, a variety of exercise program which involves a designated number of stations at which relatively hard exercises are done. Between each station an easy rhythmic exercise like walking or jogging is performed. This alternation of easy and hard work (which has already appeared in previous lessons) enables a person to work much longer than he can if performing an intense activity like handball, tennis, badminton or most other high-pressure games. Longer non-stop workouts are desirable, of course, because they lead to greater cardiovascular improvement. A standardized circuit can be designed, with ten stations for chinning, push-ups, sit-ups, leg lifts, squat jumping, vertical jumping, rope climbing, bench stepping and so on; with one or two laps of jogging required between each station. Such a circuit can then be used for competition and testing.

I. WARM–UP EXERCISES (APPROXIMATELY 25 MINUTES)

Run two laps around gym, then walk two.
Run four laps around gym, then walk two.
Run six laps around gym, then walk two.
Run eight laps around gym, then walk two.
Run ten laps around gym, then walk two.

II. CIRCUIT TRAINING (APPROXIMATELY 30 MINUTES)

a. SITTING TUCKS   **(1 MINUTE NEARLY ALL OUT)**

See Lesson One, Exercise IV f, page 107.

b. Run five laps around gym (or one quarter of a mile), then walk one lap.

c. FLUTTER KICKS   **(1 MINUTE NEARLY ALL OUT)**

See Lesson One, Exercise IV c, page 107.

d. Run five laps (or one quarter of a mile), then walk one lap.

e. ALTERNATE–SIDE LEG LIFTS   **(1 MINUTE NEARLY ALL OUT)**

See Lesson Nine, Exercise IV a, page 135.

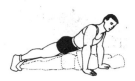

f. PUSH–UPS   **(1 MINUTE NEARLY ALL OUT)**

Starting position: Lying on floor, face down, with legs together, hands on floor next to shoulders, and fingers pointing straight ahead.

Movement: Push your body off the floor by straightening your arms so that your weight is on hands and toes. Then lower yourself until chest is barely touching floor, and raise yourself again. Repeat continuously as long as you can.

g. Run five laps (or one quarter of a mile), then walk one lap.

h. LEG LIFTS   **(1 MINUTE NEARLY ALL OUT)**

See Lesson One, Exercise IV h, page 108.

i. Run five laps (or one quarter of a mile), then walk one lap.

III. TAPERING–OFF EXERCISE (APPROXIMATELY 10 MINUTES)

Simply walk eight to ten laps, or until you feel loose and revived.

LESSON 11. 60–MINUTE MIDDLE-GEAR WORKOUT

Lesson Eleven marks the mid-point in this course and provides another good opportunity to make a progress check. If you are working on your own, you can take any of the various tests described in the first part of this book and compare the results with earlier ones. However, if you have the proper machinery and an expert operator available, you will find it enlightening to take readings of your brachial pulse wave and your blood pressure.

The Cameron Heartometer records the pulse wave in visual form, so that it can be measured by calipers (to determine the amplitude of the curve) and by a planimeter (to measure the area beneath the curve). The University of Illinois has prepared standard quantitative tables for children, for young men, and for middle-aged men and women.

Studies indicate that improvement in brachial pulse readings occur proportionately to the amount of endurance work done. This improvement shows up in waves recorded when the individual is sitting or standing at rest, but particularly during the post-exercise period. This demonstrates the tremendous value of exercise in developing cardiovascular endurance reflected in the amplitude, area and velocity of the brachial pulse wave.

I. TAKE HEARTOMETER READING—SITTING, STANDING AND AFTER RUNNING IN PLACE 180 STEPS IN ONE MINUTE.

II. WARM–UP EXERCISES (APPROXIMATELY 25 MINUTES)

See Lesson Ten, Exercise I, page 137.

III. ALTERNATE ARM–AND–LEG EXERCISES (APPROXIMATELY 30 MINUTES)

a. BENCH STEPPING   **(3 MINUTES)**

See Lesson Four, Exercise II b, page 120.

b. Work out with pulley weights, rowing machine, or medicine ball. (5 minutes)

c. Run on treadmill or repeat Bench Stepping. Then walk one lap around gym, jog two, and walk one. (3 minutes)

d. Repeat Exercise b. (5 minutes)

e. Repeat Exercise c, but walk two laps around gym, jog three, and walk two. (4 minutes)

f. Repeat Exercise b. (5 minutes)

g. Repeat Exercise c. (5 minutes)

IV. REPEAT HEARTOMETER READING

Sitting, standing and after running in place 180 steps in one minute. Compare the results with earlier reading. *

V. TAPERING–OFF EXERCISE (APPROXIMATELY 10 MINUTES)

Walk eight to ten laps around gym. Breathe deeply, stretch, and massage any tight or aching muscles. Then take a hot and cold shower, rub yourself down, and rest.

LESSON 12. 60-MINUTE MIDDLE-GEAR WORKOUT

Lesson Twelve and the following two lessons emphasize exercises and exercise routines that can be learned and practiced by the individual at home. The reason for this emphasis is to encourage you to prepare for the time when you will be on your own and may not have the convenience of a well-equipped gymnasium. You should concentrate on learning routines that you can do automatically and smoothly—combinations with enough variety to keep you from getting bored and stale. The individual circuit-training exercises in this lesson form an example of one such routine.

---

* An increase in the amplitude of the brachial pulse wave is considered a good sign, as it reflects a relative increase of the circulatory capacity. Conversely, a flat, depressed wave reflects an insufficient supply of oxygen, or a diminution of circulatory capacity. Well-trained athletes can exercise strenuously for an hour and show brachial pulse waves that are even increased in amplitude, area and velocity.

I. WARM–UP EXERCISES (APPROXIMATELY 20 MINUTES)

See Lesson Ten, Exercise I, page 137.

II. FREE EXERCISES

1. ARM AND SHOULDER EXERCISES (APPROXIMATELY 6 MINUTES)

a. CRAWL STROKES, FORWARD   (2 MINUTES)

See Lesson One, Exercise II b, page 103.

b. CRAWL STROKES, BACKWARD   (2 MINUTES)

See Lesson One, Exercise II c, page 104.

c. CROSS–BODY DOUBLE ARM CIRCLES   (2 MINUTES)

See Lesson One, Exercise II a, page 103.

2. TRUNK EXERCISES (APPROXIMATELY 9 MINUTES)

a. TORSO ROTATION, SITTING   (3 MINUTES)

See Lesson Three, Exercise III b, page 118.

b. SIT–UPS   (1 MINUTE)

See Lesson One, Exercise IV i, page 108.

c. SITTING TUCKS   (1 MINUTE)

See Lesson One, Exercise IV f, page 107.

d. LEG SPREAD   (2 MINUTES)

See Lesson Seven, Exercise IV d, page 130.

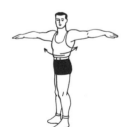

e. TORSO ROTATION, STANDING   (2 MINUTES)

Starting position: Standing, with feet about 18 inches apart, arms extended sideways.

Movement: Rotate your upper torso to the left as far as you can; then rotate right as far as you can. Repeat continuously.

III. INDIVIDUAL CIRCUIT TRAINING (APPROXIMATELY 20 MINUTES)

The following stations should be set up for the following exercises:

Station One: *Alternate-Side Leg Lifts*
                See Lesson Nine, Exercise IV a, page 135.

Station Two: *Push-Ups*
                 See Lesson Ten, Exercise II f, page 138.

Station Three: *Sitting Tucks*
                 See Lesson One, Exercise IV f, page 107.

Station Four: *Vertical Jumps*
                 See Lesson Two, Exercise IV f, page 115.

Start at Station One, do exercise 10 times (5 on each side); run one lap around gym; go to Station Two, do exercise 10 times; run lap around gym; go to Station Three, etc. On second round do exercises 15 times; on third round, 20 times; on fourth round, 25 times. (If you are performing exercises at home, run in place between each station.) Walk, stretch, and breathe to recover.

IV. REPEAT EXERCISES 1 AND 2 ABOVE (OPTIONAL)

V. REPEAT INDIVIDUAL CIRCUIT TRAINING (OPTIONAL)

VI. TAPERING–OFF EXERCISE (APPROXIMATELY 5 MINUTES)

Walk around gym for about 5 minutes, stretch, shake your limbs, breathe to recover. Take a hot and cold shower, rub yourself down, and rest.

LESSON 13.   60–MINUTE MIDDLE–GEAR WORKOUT

In Lesson Thirteen you will continue to get practice in self-directed workouts. The purpose of this lesson is to teach routines which can be carried out alone or in a small group. The general plan is to warm up for twenty to thirty minutes with special exercises; then to do three training routines to emphasize (1) arm and back strength, (2) leg and body strength, and (3) interval training running; and finally to do tapering-off exercises.

I. SELF–DIRECTED WARM–UP EXERCISES (APPROXIMATELY 25 MINUTES)

Spend the warm-up period working on a bicycle, a treadmill, or doing a walk-jog-walk-jog routine.

II. SELF–DIRECTED HARD EXERCISES (APPROXIMATELY 35 MIN-
UTES)

1. Arm and Back Work

a. MEDICINE BALL EXERCISES   **(10 MINUTES)**

See Lesson Seven, Exercise IV b, page 130.

2. Leg and Body Work

a. BENCH–STEPPING EXERCISE   **(1 MINUTE)**

See Lesson Four, Exercise II b, page 120. Lead with left foot.

b. Stretch, bend, breathe deeply and shake yourself out. (1 minute)

c. BENCH–STEPPING EXERCISE   **(1 MINUTE)**

Lead with right foot.

d. PUSH–UPS   **(1 MINUTE)**

See Lesson Ten, Exercise II f, page 138.

e. BENCH–STEPPING EXERCISE   **(1 MINUTE)**

Lead with left foot.

f. ALTERNATE–SIDE LEG LIFTS   **(30 ON EACH SIDE)**

See Lesson Nine, Exercise IV a, page 135.

g. BENCH–STEPPING EXERCISE   **(1 MINUTE)**

Lead with right foot.

h. LEG LIFTS   **(1 MINUTE)**

See Lesson One, Exercise IV h, page 108.

i. BENCH–STEPPING EXERCISE   **(1 MINUTE)**

Lead with left foot.

j. FLUTTER KICKS   **(30 ON FRONT, AND 30 ON BACK)**

See Lesson One, Exercise IV c, page 107.

k. BENCH–STEPPING EXERCISE   **(1 MINUTE)**

Lead with right foot.

l. SIT–UPS   **(1 MINUTE)**

See Lesson One, Exercise IV i, page 108.

m. BENCH–STEPPING EXERCISE   (1 MINUTE)

Lead with left foot.

3. Interval Training

Jog two laps around gym, then walk one.
Jog four laps, then walk one.
Jog six laps, then walk one.
Run eight laps, then walk two.
Run ten laps, then walk ten.

III. TAPERING–OFF EXERCISE (APPROXIMATELY 5 MINUTES)

Walk around gym for about five minutes, breathe deeply, stretch, and shake out your limbs. Massage any tight muscles. Take a hot and cold shower, and rest.

LESSON 14.   60–MINUTE MIDDLE–GEAR WORKOUT

Lesson Fourteen contains a series of exercises which do not require special equipment like pulley weights, medicine balls or rowing machines. They are free exercises which, except for the warm-up and tapering-off phases, require only a little floor space to perform. They are emphasized here as further examples of exercises you can do at home and independent of a class.

I. WARM–UP EXERCISES (APPROXIMATELY 30 MINUTES)

At moderate speed jog half a mile (or run in place for 5 minutes). Walk one quarter mile, all the while stretching and flexing arms and breathing deeply.
At three-quarter speed, sprint 100 yards (or run in place rapidly for 20 seconds).
Jog one-quarter mile slowly, breathing deeply (or run in place rapidly for 20 seconds).
At three-quarter speed, sprint 200 yards (or run in place rapidly for 30 seconds).
Jog one-quarter mile slowly, breathing deeply.
At three-quarter speed, sprint 300 yards (or run in place rapidly for 40 seconds).
Jog one-quarter mile slowly, breathing deeply.

At three-quarter speed, sprint 400 yards (or run in place rapidly for 50 seconds).

Walk one-quarter mile, all the while stretching and flexing arms, and occasionally bouncing up and down in a squatting position.

II. ARM AND SHOULDER EXERCISES (APPROXIMATELY 5 MINUTES)

See Lesson Three, Section II, pages 116–17.

III. FLEXIBILITY EXERCISES (APPROXIMATELY 5 MINUTES)

a. ARM STRETCHES AND BODY TURNS (1 MINUTE)

See Lesson Two, Exercise I b, page 110.

b. ARM SWINGING, FORWARD AND BACKWARD IN OPPOSITION (1 MINUTE)

See Lesson One, Exercise II e, page 104.

c. TRUNK BENDS (1 MINUTE)

See Lesson One, Exercise IV e, page 107.

d. CROSS–BODY FLOOR TOUCHES (1 MINUTE)

See Lesson One, Exercise III a, page 105.

e. TRUNK FLEXIONS AND ROTATIONS (1 MINUTE)

See Lesson Two, Exercise I h, page 111.

IV. WAIST EXERCISES (APPROXIMATELY 5 MINUTES)

a. SIT–UPS (DO 60)

See Lesson One, Exercise IV i, page 108.

b. TORSO ROTATION, SITTING (DO 30 EACH WAY)

See Lesson Three, Exercise III b, page 118.

c. V–SITS (1 MINUTE)

See Lesson Seven, Exercise IV f, page 131.

d. CHEST LIFTS (DO 30)

See Lesson One, Exercise IV g, page 107.

e. ALTERNATE–SIDE LEG LIFTS (1 MINUTE)

See Lesson Nine, Exercise IV a, page 135.

V. HARD BODY EXERCISES (APPROXIMATELY 5 MINUTES)

a. PUSH–UPS   (DO 20)

See Lesson Ten, Exercise II f, page 138.

b. LEG LIFTS   (2 MINUTES)

See Lesson One, Exercise IV h, page 108.

c. SIT–UPS   (2 MINUTES)

See Lesson One, Exercise IV i, page 108.

VI. LEG EXERCISES (APPROXIMATELY 5 MINUTES)

a. HOPPING ON ALTERNATE FEET   (1 MINUTE)

See Lesson One, Exercise V e, page 109.

b. TOE–HEEL PRANCE   (1 LAP AROUND GYM)

See Lesson Five, Exercise III b, page 122.

c. RUNNING IN PLACE   (1 MINUTE)

Lift feet at least 12 inches off the floor.

d. Skip sideways one lap around gym, then reverse direction and skip sideways one lap.

VII. TAPERING–OFF EXERCISES (APPROXIMATELY 10 MINUTES)

Walk and jog eight to ten laps around gym, breathing deeply, stretching, kicking, and shaking. Take a hot and cold shower, rub yourself down, and rest.

LESSON 15. 60–MINUTE MIDDLE–GEAR WORKOUT

Lesson Fifteen marks the beginning of the transition to high-gear exercising. Although the lesson remains essentially a middle-gear workout, you will find that we have introduced an important ingredient of high-gear exercising, namely exercises involving team competition, which in this case take the form of relay races.

The relay race can be arranged in many ways. It can cover a

course that travels in circular laps, that shuttles back and forth across a given distance, or that describes some special pattern like a figure eight. It can require the participant to run, walk, hop, crawl, dribble a basketball and so on. The important thing for you is that it combines individual performance of a certain feat with team competition. It is a device for motivating you to exert yourself harder than you might if you were simply trying to perform a certain exercise a certain number of times. Just why the element of competition is important to high-gear exercising will be explained in a later lesson.

I. WARM–UP EXERCISES (APPROXIMATELY 15 MINUTES)

Run two laps around gym, then walk one lap.
Run four laps around gym, then walk one lap.
Run six laps around gym, then walk one lap.
Run eight laps around gym, then walk one lap.
Run ten laps around gym, then walk two laps.

II. TEAM RELAY–RACING COMPETITION

The instructor should divide the class into two teams, with the same number of people on each team. The teams should complete the relay course one at a time, racing against the clock. The team with the lowest time wins, and the individual with the lowest time wins.

Run two laps around the gym; then hop the length of the gym on the left foot and one length of the gym on the right foot; then walk two laps around the gym. When you have finished, touch the hand of the next person on your team, who will then run the same course.

III. INDIVIDUAL CIRCUIT TRAINING

The following stations should be set up for the following exercises:

Station One: *V-Sit*
                 See Lesson Seven, Exercise IV f, page 131.

Station Two: *Flutter Kicks, on Back*
                 See Lesson One, Exercise IV c, page 107.

Station Three: *Flutter Kicks, on Front*
                 See Lesson One, Exercise IV c, page 107.

Station Four: *Stick Body* (with partner)

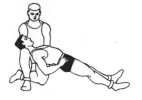

Starting position: Reclining, with head resting on partner's knee or hands, feet on floor, arms folded across stomach.

Movement: Hold your body rigidly straight for 30 seconds.

Start at Station One. Do exercise for 30 seconds.

Run one lap around gym.

Go to Station Two. Do exercise 100 times.

Run one lap around gym.

Go to Station Three. Do exercise 100 times.

Run one lap around gym.

Go to Station Four. Do exercise for 30 seconds.

Run one lap around gym.

Go back to Station One.

On second round do exercises for 40 seconds or 150 times; on third round do exercises 50 seconds or 200 times; on fourth round do exercises 60 seconds or 250 times.

IV. TAPERING–OFF EXERCISES (APPROXIMATELY 10 MINUTES)

Jog five times around gym, then walk five laps. Breathe deeply, stretch, kick, and shake out limbs. Massage tight or sore muscles. Take hot and cold shower, rub-down, and rest.

LESSON 16.   60–MINUTE MIDDLE–GEAR WORKOUT

Lesson Sixteen continues the preparation for high-gear exercising. The feature of the lesson is a set of exercises that we call double-dose exercises. These are simply sets of exercises interrupted by very brief rest periods. Their significant feature is that each pair exercises the same set of muscles—sometimes in two or more different ways, and with progressively increased intensity. This distinguishes them from earlier paired sets of exercises, which tend not to exercise the same set of muscles together. As you can see, we are working gradually toward workout periods of maximum intensity of effort, and trying to prepare you for the different ways by which maximum intensity can be achieved.

I. WARM–UP EXERCISES (APPROXIMATELY 20 MINUTES)

Preliminary warm-up should consist of bench stepping, walking, while practicing arm and chest movements, and body bending, twisting and stretching. By this point you should be familiar enough with the various exercises to select the ones that you find most effective. Be sure to keep exercising continuously.

II. DOUBLE–DOSE EXERCISES (APPROXIMATELY 30 MINUTES)

These exercises can be performed individually or in a group. The instructor should explain the plan for the entire workout, lead each exercise himself, and explain as the work progresses what the purpose of each exercise is, i.e., which part of the body is affected and what the benefit is.

a. Jog in place for 2 minutes, stop and take 10 deep breaths;
   Then do 30 *Sitting Tucks.*
   For Sitting Tucks, See Lesson One, Exercise IV f, page 107.

b. Walk one lap around gym, breathing, stretching, and shaking to recover.

c. *Butterfly Arm Strokes* for 2 minutes

   See Lesson One, Exercise II f, page 104, stop and take 10 deep breaths;
   Then do 30 *Sitting Frog Kicks.*

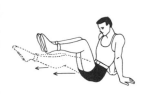

Starting position: Sitting, with hands on floor beside hips and legs extended.

Movement: Draw both feet up simultaneously until your heels are almost touching your buttocks. Then thrust them *apart* and forward, and bring them together again.

d. Walk one lap around gym, repeating recuperative procedures.

e. Jog in place for 2 minutes, stop and take 10 deep breaths;
   Do 10 *Push-Ups.*
   For Push-Ups, see Lesson Ten, Exercise II f, page 138.

f. Walk one lap around gym, repeating recuperative procedures.

g. Do 100 *Flutter Kicks, on Back* See Lesson One, Exercise IV c, page 107, take 10 deep breaths;
Do 100 *Flutter Kicks, on Front,* take 10 deep breaths;
Do 100 *Side Leg Kicks* on each side.
(See Lesson One, Exercise IV b, page 106.)
Take 10 deep breaths, walk around gym one lap, jog around gym one lap.

h. AGILITY RUN

Starting position: Standing, at one end of a line of four chairs or stools placed 10 feet apart.

Movement: At signal, run at top speed zig-zagging between the chairs, around the last chair, and back again.

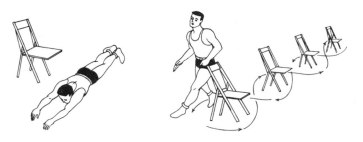

Then walk two laps, repeating recuperative procedures.

Repeat agility run and 2 laps until you have run through the course 5 times.

III. TAPERING–OFF EXERCISES (APPROXIMATELY 10 MINUTES)

Walk and jog, breathing, stretching, shaking and kicking, until you feel rested.

LESSON 17.   60–MINUTE MIDDLE–GEAR WORKOUT

Lesson Seventeen—the last middle-gear workout—develops the system of multiple-dose exercises further. In the following workout, you will perform the same exercise *four* times for increasingly long intervals. By the time you are on the fourth round of each exercise you should be working close to maximum speed and effort.

I. WARM–UP EXERCISES (APPROXIMATELY 25 MINUTES)

a. Alternately walk and jog one half-mile around the gym or a field.

b. Perform stretching, bending, twisting, deep breathing and arm exercises for about fifteen minutes.

II. RHYTHMICAL ENDURANCE EXERCISES (APPROXIMATELY 30 MINUTES)

You may perform these exercises by yourself or with a group. If you are in a class, the instructor should explain the plan for the entire period, lead each exercise himself, and explain as the work progresses what the purpose of each exercise is, i.e., which part of the body is affected and what the benefit is.

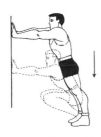

a. LEANING SQUATS

Starting position: Leaning, with hands against wall and feet at least 3 feet from base of wall.

Movement: Squat down until you are in a three-quarter squat. Then return to a standing position.

First Round: 15 times
Second Round: 30 times
Third Round: 45 times
Fourth Round: 60 times

Between each round breathe deeply and stretch—for one minute.

b. SITTING TUCKS

See Lesson One, Exercise IV f, page 107.

First Round: 15 times
Second Round: 30 times
Third Round: 45 times
Fourth Round: 60 times

Between each round breathe deeply and stretch—for one minute.

c. FLUTTER KICKS, ON FRONT

See Lesson One, Exercise IV c, page 107.

First Round: 50 times   Between each round breathe deeply and
Second Round: 100 times   stretch—for one minute.
Third Round: 200 times
Fourth Round: 300 times

d. SIDE LEG KICKS

See Lesson One, Exercise IV b, page 106.

First Round: Short, narrow kicks—50 times left, 50 times right.
Second Round: High kicks—50 times left, 50 times right.
Third Round: Short kicks—100 times left, 100 times right.
Fourth Round: High kicks—100 times left, 100 times right.

e. RUNNING LAPS

First Round: Run three laps, walk two laps.
Second Round: Run six laps, walk two laps.
Third Round: Run nine laps, walk two laps.
Fourth Round: Run twelve laps, walk two laps.

III. TAPERING–OFF EXERCISES

Walk around gym using recuperative procedures until you have recovered. Shower and rub yourself down with towel. Rest and recover.

LESSON 18.   60-MINUTE HIGH-GEAR WORKOUT

From Lesson Eighteen until the end of the course you will be working at high-gear exercises. Your basic objective in these exercises should be to push yourself as near as possible to the limits of your strength and endurance.

In recent years, we have learned a great deal about how far a person can push himself. Through the courageous feats of people like Dr. Roger Bannister, we have discovered that the human body can stand much more punishment than was once thought. We know that everyone has a point beyond which he cannot make himself perform, but we also know that this point is more psychological than physiological. Unless a person is unusually motivated, he will cease to be able to push himself long before he has reached the end of his physical limits. The body has not really been extended—that is, you are not really going "all out"—until you feel nauseous, develop cramps and shows signs of losing your coordination. Even when these symptoms appear, you are far from the point where real harm can occur.

The object of these high-gear exercises is to push back the point of psychological exhaustion, and get you closer to actual physical exhaustion. This is the only real way to develop first-class strength and endurance.

I. WARM–UP EXERCISES (APPROXIMATELY 20 MINUTES)

Run two laps around gym, then walk one.
Run four laps, then walk one.
Run six laps, then walk one.
Run eight laps, then walk one.
Run ten laps, then walk for three minutes.

II. ALL–OUT EXERCISES (APPROXIMATELY 30 MINUTES)

Perform the following exercises at top speed and to the absolute limits of your strength and endurance. In each case record the number of exercises you were able to do.

a. SITTING TUCKS

See Lesson One, Exercise IV f, page 107.

b. Walk slowly around gym once, breathing deeply, stretching and shaking out your arms and legs.

c. FLUTTER KICKS, FRONT AND BACK

See Lesson One, Exercise IV c, page 107.

d. Walk slowly around gym once, breathing deeply, stretching and shaking out your arms and legs. Bend and touch the floor a few times.

e. PUSH–UPS

See Lesson Ten, Exercise II f, page 138.

f. Walk slowly around gym once, breathing deeply, stretching and shaking your arms and legs.

g. SIDE LEG KICKS, ON BOTH SIDES

See Lesson One, Exercise IV b, page 106.

h. Walk slowly around gym once, breathing deeply, stretching and shaking out your arms and legs.

i. SQUAT JUMPS

See Lesson Six, Exercise IV b, page 127.

j. Walk slowly around gym once, breathing deeply, stretching and shaking out your arms and legs.

III. TAPERING–OFF EXERCISES (APPROXIMATELY 20 MINUTES)

a. Jog five laps around gym, slowly.

b. Walk five laps around gym, breathing deeply and stretching.

c. Jog one lap around gym very slowly. Shake and relax.

d. Walk, breathe deeply and stretch until almost recovered.

e. Massage calves and thighs, and take a hot shower followed by a cold shower. Then rub yourself down briskly.

When you have finished, lie down and relax as fully as possible for twenty minutes. After very hard work, it is a good idea to wait an hour before eating.

LESSON 19. 90–MINUTE HIGH–GEAR WORKOUT

In the introduction to the previous lesson, we said that the main object of these high-gear workouts is to push back the point where you become exhausted. To do this, you must be psychologically stimulated to perform extraordinarily hard. These lessons are designed to provide such stimulation in a number of ways. If you are going through these workouts in a formal class led by an instructor, you will be motivated a great deal by performing in a group, in front of a critical person. It is surprising how much easier it is to extend yourself physically if you are working in a group "by the numbers." A group provides company and a little competition, and competition is an especially effective way of prodding a person to exert himself further than he might go on his own. For this reason particular relay races and other competitive gimmicks have been included in some of the lessons. You can compete against yourself, too. That is why it is suggested that you record the number of exercises you do. It gives you a mark to shoot for, to see if you can beat your previous record and steadily improve yourself.

It is remarkable how effective these psychological goads have proved in the past. After a few months it becomes possible for most adults to go through a workout including as many as five or six all-out exercises. At the University of Illinois Fitness Center, we have put more than 50,000 people through an eight-battery workout involving four strength exercises, three flexibility exercises, one agility exercise, one power exercise, one breath-holding exercise, and five endurance exercises. Not one person has suffered any ill effects from this rigorous routine.

I. WARM–UP EXERCISES (APPROXIMATELY 20 MINUTES)

Run two laps, walk one.
Run four laps, walk one.
Run six laps, walk one.
Run ten laps, walk for three minutes.

II. ALL–OUT EXERCISES (APPROXIMATELY 30 MINUTES)

Perform the following exercises at top speed and to the absolute limits of your strength and endurance. In each case, record the number of exercises you were able to do or the length of time it took you to perform the exercise.

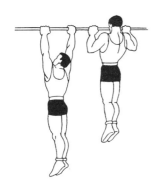

a. CHIN–UPS

Starting position: Hanging by hands from horizontal bar with knuckles toward your face, arms straight, legs straight, feet off the ground.

Movement: Pull yourself up by bending your arms until your chin is above the level of the top of the bar. Then lower yourself until your arms are straight again. Repeat continuously as many times as possible.

b. Walk slowly around gym once, breathing deeply, kicking, shaking and stretching.

c. VERTICAL JUMPS

See Lesson Two, Exercise IV f, page 115.

d. Walk slowly around gym once, breathing deeply, kicking, shaking and stretching.

e. SIT–UPS

See Lesson One, Exercise IV i, page 108.

f. Walk slowly around gym once, breathing deeply, kicking, shaking and stretching.

g. STICK BODY

See Lesson Fifteen, Exercise III, Station Four, page 148.

h. Walk slowly around gym once, breathing deeply, kicking, shaking and stretching.

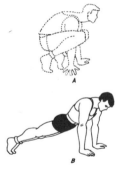

i. BURPEE

Starting position: Standing, with feet together and arms at side.

Movement: Squat, place your hands on the floor, kick your legs back so that you are in the front leaning rest position, bring your legs forward so that you are back in a squat, and stand up. Repeat as fast as possible for 20 seconds.

j. Walk slowly around gym once, breathing deeply, kicking, shaking and stretching.

k. PUSH–UPS

See Lesson Ten, Exercise II f, page 138.

l. Walk slowly around gym once, breathing deeply, kicking, shaking and stretching.

III. RELAXATION EXERCISES (APPROXIMATELY 3 MINUTES)

a. Jog around gym twice.

b. Walk around gym once, breathing deeply, kicking, shaking and and stretching.

IV. ALL–OUT EXERCISES (APPROXIMATELY 30 MINUTES)

Repeat Section II.

V. TAPERING–OFF EXERCISES (APPROXIMATELY 15 MINUTES)

a. Slowly jog five laps around gym, staying flat-footed and relaxing.

b. Walk five laps around gym; breathe deeply and stretch.

c. Walk, breathe deeply and stretch until recovered. Do *Upside-Down Bicycle* (without stall bar), bracing your back with your hands against the small of your back, elbows braced on the floor. See Lesson Seven, Exercise IV i, page 131.

d. Massage calves and thighs, and take a hot shower, followed by a cold shower.

When you have finished, lie down and relax as fully as possible for twenty minutes. Remember that it is a good idea not to eat for an hour.

LESSON **20.**   90–MINUTE HIGH–GEAR WORKOUT

Lesson Twenty brings you well into the high-gear level workouts. Now that you have adapted to this strenuous level of exercising, you may want to see how your physical condition compares with that of other people of your age and general circumstances. There are many tests available to serve this purpose. We have already mentioned the eighteen-item Motor-Fitness Test which appears in the first part of this book, and there is also our Standard Test of General Physical Fitness (See Chapter Two, pages 37–40) which you may want to take again at this point. Cardiovascular tests are also important and enlightening, but it is wisest to take these after consultation with your doctor. In addition, there are standard tests of your ability to stand on a balance beam, do push-ups, chin-ups, squat jumps and so on. Then there are tests used by the Armed Forces, by YMCA groups and by police groups. It might be most enlightening for you to see how you stack up in these various tests. They help you to understand your potential energy level and athletic ability.

I. WARM–UP EXERCISES (APPROXIMATELY 20 MINUTES)

Run two laps, walk one.
Run four laps, walk one.
Run six laps, walk one.
Run eight laps, walk one.
Run ten laps, walk three laps, then breathe, shake and stretch.

II. ALL–OUT EXERCISES (APPROXIMATELY 30 MINUTES)

Perform the following exercises at top speed and to the absolute limits of your strength and endurance. In each case, record the number of exercises that you were able to do or the length of time you were able to perform the exercise.

a. V–SITS

See Lesson Seven, Exercise IV f, page 131.

b. Walk slowly around gym once, breathing deeply, shaking and stretching.

c. ALTERNATE–SIDE LEG LIFTS

See Lesson Nine, Exercise IV a, page 135.

d. Walk slowly around gym once, breathing deeply, shaking and stretching.

e. CHEST LIFTS

See Lesson One, Exercise IV g, page 107.

f. Walk slowly around gym once, breathing deeply, shaking and stretching.

g. AGILITY RUN

See Lesson Sixteen, Exercise II h, page 150.

h. Walk slowly around gym once, breathing deeply, shaking and stretching.

i. JUMPING JACKS

See Lesson One, Exercise II h, page 105.

j. Walk slowly around gym once, breathing deeply, shaking and stretching.

III. OUTDOOR RUNNING EXERCISE (APPROXIMATELY 7 MINUTES)

Run down a flight of stairs, run outdoors and run about 600 yards. Then run indoors and upstairs. When you have finished, don't stop suddenly, but taper off by walking and breathing deeply.

IV. RELAXATION EXERCISES (APPROXIMATELY 4 MINUTES)

a. Jog around the gym twice.

b. Walk around the gym twice.

V. ALL–OUT EXERCISES (APPROXIMATELY 30 MINUTES)

Repeat Section II.

VI. TAPERING–OFF EXERCISES (APPROXIMATELY 15 MINUTES)

a. Jog slowly five laps around gym.

b. Walk slowly five laps around gym.

c. Jog slowly one lap around gym.

d. Walk, breathing deeply and stretching, until recovered. Lie on your back, breathe deeply and relax.

e. Take a hot shower, then a cold one.

When you have finished, lie down and relax as fully as possible for twenty minutes. Remember that it is a good idea not to eat for an hour.

LESSON 21. HIGH-GEAR ENDURANCE WORKOUT

Perhaps the most important ingredient of physical fitness is endurance, the human capacity to stand pain, distress and fatigue over a lengthy period of time. Good endurance is the result of a combination of will power, a strong and tough central nervous system, muscular fitness and cardiovascular fitness. Your power of endurance is possibly one of the more sensitive gauges to your general condition, and the most tangible evidence of any gains in physical fitness you may have made.

Lesson Twenty-one contains ten endurance workouts which will serve both as tests of your endurance and exercises to help further develop your powers of endurance. The ten exercises should *not* be attempted all together as a single workout. As you will see, one exercise alone will constitute a day's work.

I. 100–MILE RUN

Work at becoming a member of a 100-Mile Running Club by running 100 cumulative miles in two weeks. Only whole miles count.

II. MARATHON SWIM

Swim the equivalent of 26 miles in a swimming pool.

III. 3–MILE MEDLEY

Run a mile, row a mile (or the equivalent on a rowing machine—about 10 minutes of rowing) and swim a mile continuously.

IV. ALL–OUT EXERCISES

Exercise continually for an hour using all-out exercises. Be sure to include warm-up and tapering-off stages.

V. TWENTY–MILE HIKE

Hike 20 miles in one day.

VI. LAP RUNNING

Over a three-week period:

a. Run a lap and walk a lap. Repeat 20 times. Do this for one week.

b. Run two laps and walk one; run four laps and walk one; run six laps and walk one; run eight laps and walk one; run ten laps and walk one.
Do this for one week.

c. Run ten laps and walk one; run eight faster laps and walk one; run six faster laps and walk one; run four fast laps and walk one; sprint two laps and walk ten.

VII. MORE ALL–OUT EXERCISES

Over a one-hour period, perform the following exercises at the peak of your ability:
Chin the bar, do push-ups, do sitting tucks, do side leg raises on both sides and do squat jumps.

VIII. TREADMILL WALK

For 30 minutes walk on a treadmill set on an 8.6 per cent grade at a speed of 3½ mph.

IX. TREADMILL JOG

Jog for 15 minutes on a treadmill set on an 8.6 per cent grade at a speed of 5 mph.

X. ENDURANCE THROWING AND RUNNING

Throw a javelin, boomerang, medicine ball, football or baseball as far as you can. Recover object thrown and return to throwing place at a top-speed run. Repeat 50 times in a single workout.

LESSON 22.   HIGH–GEAR TREADMILL WORKOUT

If continued long enough, walking on a graded treadmill is one of the best all-around exercises for reducing fat and getting in shape. A thirty-minute walk will serve to stimulate your circulation and cause full and deep respiration, as well as free perspiration.

While walking up a long hill or walking up and down stairs is just as effective as walking on a treadmill, a treadmill has certain advantages, among them the fact that it is stationary and usually located where you are doing your training. It should be set on an 8.6 per cent grade, at a speed of three-and-one-half miles per hour for people of medium height and four miles per hour for taller people.

In this lesson you will find a useful set of exercises that you can do on a treadmill. If the model that you are using is equipped with a waist strap, secure it so that you arms will be free.

I. TREADMILL EXERCISES AND PROCEDURES

a. With the treadmill set at a pace equivalent to a brisk walk, note the time and walk in an ordinary manner for 10 minutes.

b. Now, as you walk, lift your knees a bit higher, and flex your arms —up on one step and down on the next. At the same time, try to breathe deeply. Continue walking in this manner for 5 minutes.

c. Now walk in an ordinary fashion for 5 more minutes.

d. Now, without breaking your stride, swing both arms in full circles. Continue walking in this manner for 2 minutes.

e. Now, continue swinging your arms, hard, first holding them straight, then bending them at the elbows so that your fists rest on your chest. Continue walking in this manner for 5 minutes.

f. Now, raise your arms straight up in the air and breathe deeply. Continue walking in this manner for 5 minutes, then shake and stretch until you have recovered.

Section II

SPECIAL EXERCISES
FOR VARIOUS PARTS
OF THE BODY

Introduction

The following section includes exercises which are recommended for specific parts of the body. They are included for the benefit of people who need to work on one or more particularly deficient areas of their body.

Once you have decided that you have a certain deficiency, either from your own observation or as the result of consultation with a physician or an instructor, we recommend that in addition to your regular workout period you devote fifteen minutes to these special exercises.

The areas covered by the following exercises include the abdominal muscles, the muscles of the buttocks, the waist, the lower back region, the feet and legs, and the upper body, shoulders and neck. Some of the exercises will be new to you, while many others will be the same as those you encountered in the progressive workouts.

1. Special Exercises for the Abdominal Muscles

Since the muscles of the stomach are among the first to be affected by lack of activity, and since the development of middle-aged "bulge" is one of the most unsightly aspects of physical decline, many people are particularly interested in exercises for the abdominal muscles.

This concern is justifiable, for the shape of the stomach muscles affects more than just appearance. The condition of the abdominal muscles influences the flow of blood through the big abdominal veins that lead back to the heart. Poor abdominal condition, coupled with flaccid leg veins, usually results in pooling of the blood in the large veins of the legs and lower abdomen, especially in sitting or standing postures. This is most undesirable, for it affects both the supply of nutrition to the abdominal region and the efficiency of the entire circulatory system.

Running, bench stepping, knee-bend squats, deep breathing, the application of cold packs, or squeezing and kneading the abdomen, serve either to force blood out of the mesenteries and abdominal veins or to activate the sympathetic nervous system to draw the blood back into the central circulatory system.

Rhythmical contraction of the abdominal muscles (in leg lifts and sit-ups), alternated with bending and squeezing of the viscera, results in improved circulation and better muscle tone. Deep and forceful breathing should accompany such exercises.

Cold bathing will also help to move pooled blood into general circulation, as will underwater swimming. All exercises should be followed by deep breathing.

The following exercises will provide you with a progressive program for strengthening the stomach muscles.

FIVE SETS OF PROGRESSIVE ABDOMINAL EXERCISES

	EASY	MODERATE	HARD
I.	Lying on your back, with hands behind neck, lift and bend fully each leg alternately. (Do 20 bends with each leg.)	Lying on your back, with hands behind neck, lift and bend both legs simultaneously. (Do 20 times.)	Lying on your back, with hands behind neck, lift both legs simultaneously to vertical position. (Do 20 lifts.)
II.	Lying on your back, with hands at sides and legs held down, do a half sit-up by raising your trunk to a 45 degree angle. (Do 20 times.)	Lying on your back, with hands at sides and legs held down, do a full sit-up by bringing your trunk up to a vertical position. (Do 20 times.)	Lying on your back, with hands behind neck and legs held down, do a full sit-up. (Do 20 times.)
III.	Lying on your back, with hands at sides and legs free, do a half sit-up. (Do 20 times.)	Lying on your back, with hands at sides and legs free, do a full sit-up. (Do 20 times.)	Lying on your back, with hands at sides and legs free, do *rapid* full sit-ups. (Repeat until moderately tired.)
IV.	Lying on your back, with hands behind neck and legs free, do a half sit-up. (Do 20 times.)	Lying on your back, with hands behind neck and legs free, do a full sit-up. (Do 20 times.)	Lying on your back, with hands behind neck and legs free, do *rapid* sit-ups. (Repeat until moderately tired.)
V.	Lying on your back, with hands behind neck and legs free, do as many sit-ups as you can.	Lying on your back, with hands behind neck, do full leg lifts. (Do as many as you can.)	Lying on your back, with hands behind neck and legs free, do leg lifts and sit-ups alternately. (Continue as long as you can.)

2. Special Exercises for the Gluteal (Buttock) Muscles

One of the first casualties of the inactive middle-age years are the gluteal muscles of the buttocks. As a result of long periods of sitting or standing still, they tend to soften and lose their tone. The results are both unattractive and unhealthy.

One particular result of this deterioration is the loosening of the joint between the hip bone (*ilium*) and the lower spine (*sacrum*), which are held together by the gluteal muscles. Since there are no ligaments across the posterior surface of this particular joint, muscle tone is necessary to hold it together. Weakening of the joint can result in irritation of the nerves around the joint, a complication which can be very painful. Sacroiliac strain is another familiar result of weak gluteal muscles; it usually occurs when a person picks up a heavy object by bending over from the waist without bending his knees.

The typical middle-aged person should make a special effort to keep his gluteal muscles in good shape, especially if he leads an inactive life.

There are a number of exercises which are very useful for toning up the glutei. If you are an inactive person you will probably find that when you stand in a relaxed position your pelvis tilts forward and downward, causing your stomach to protrude and your spine to curve. Consciously tilting the pelvis backward and upward serves to straighten the spine, pull the stomach in, and tense the gluteal muscles. Place your back against the wall or the floor and flatten your lower spine until you can feel it touching the surface. Hold this position for ten seconds and release it. Repeat this movement again and again. It will teach you what it feels like to tilt your pelvis correctly, and help to strengthen your buttock muscles.

Another effective exercise is done by standing on tiptoe, tensing the glutei vigorously, and hitting your buttocks with your fist.

Sprinting, running and running in place are other good ways to strengthen the muscles in your buttocks as well as to remove excess fat from the seat and the upper thighs. Cycling, skiing and long-distance running are all helpful activities for the sedentary middle-aged person.

3. Special Exercises for the Muscles in the Waist

The waist muscles are used to bend the upper body sideways, in all twisting movements of trunk on the pelvis and the pelvis on the legs. The deep muscles known as the *quadratus lumborum,* which attach the pelvis to the spine, are involved in all of these movements. Normally very strong, these muscles can be seriously weakened by years of disuse. Ordinary strolling and standing are not adequate to maintain their fitness.

Activities which condition the waist muscles include boxing (or striking out with the fist and arm), wrestling, shot-putting, tennis, bowling, throwing a baseball or javelin, swimming the crawl stroke, and the frog kick used in the breast stroke. These are but a few of the activities which require the use of the lateral twisting muscles. The list also illustrates how important these muscles are in sports.

The following exercises and procedures are specifically recommended for strengthening the waist muscles:

I. V–SIT, SCISSORS KICK

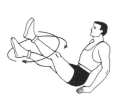

Starting position: Sitting, with trunk and legs lifted off the floor so that body forms a V, hands on floor.

Movement: Holding the V-sit position, spread your legs apart, bring them together, cross them over and under each other, and return them to the starting position. Repeat continuously at the rate of about 60 a minute.

II. SIDEWAYS SIT–UPS

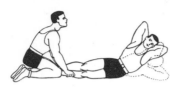

Starting position: Lying on side, with legs held down by a partner or some piece of furniture or a set of stall bars, and with fingers laced behind neck.

Movement: Raise your body sideways from the waist as high as you can. Try to stay on your side as much as possible. Repeat 10 to 30 times, then turn over and repeat on other side.

III. SIDE LEG KICKS, SHORT

See Progressive Course, Lesson One, Exercise IV b, page 106. Do 20 to 50 on each side.

IV. SIDE LEANING LEG LIFTS

See Progressive Course, Lesson Six, Exercise IV c, page 127.

V. CROSS–OVER HIP ROLL

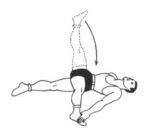

Starting position: Lying on back, with legs extended straight and arms at sides.

Movement: Raise your right leg to a vertical position, roll over onto your left hip and, keeping both legs straight, touch your right toe to your left hand, then return to starting position. Repeat same movement to right side. Do 10 to 50 times on each side.

VI. ALTERNATE–SIDE LEG LIFTS

See Progressive Course, Lesson Nine, Exercise IV a, page 135.

VII. TRUNK WIGWAG ON FRONT

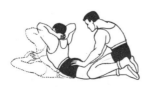

Starting position: Lying face down, with hands behind neck and legs held down by partner, furniture, or stall bars.

Movement: Raise your chest and head off the floor and wigwag your trunk to the right and to the left repeatedly.

VIII. TRUNK WIGWAG ON BACK

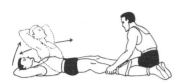

Starting position: Lying on back, with hands behind neck and legs held down by partner, furniture, or stall bars.

Movement: Raise your trunk to a half-sitting position and wigwag to the right and to the left repeatedly.

4. Special Exercises for the Lower Back Region

The lower part of your spine is held in place by a series of muscle groups which attach the spine and the legs to the pelvis. Unless these muscles are kept in good condition, they weaken, allowing the spine to be displaced forward, pinching the nerves and blood vessels in the immediate vicinity. The result is fatigue of the lower back, poor circulation and sometimes even severe pain, as well as sacroiliac strain.

Active, well-conditioned athletes rarely complain of such pain, even when they are in their thirties, forties and fifties, whereas sedentary people very frequently complain of such trouble.

Exercises which restore the fitness of the lower back muscles are those which contract the hip and back extensors through hyperextension of the back, as opposed to forward trunk flexion. One such exercise is done by lying face down on the floor, with the head raised, the hands placed beneath the thighs and the back in a slightly arched position. The legs are then kicked up and down as they are in swimming the flutter kick. A slight variation of this exercise is to lift both legs simultaneously, so as to increase the arch of the back.

The lateral muscles (*quadratus lumborum*) which connect the spine to the pelvis can be exercised by standing and kneeling rotations of the trunk on the pelvis. More vigorous training of the lower back can be achieved by working with a partner, or by placing the feet beneath the lowest rung of a set of stall bars, under a piece of furniture like a davenport, or even under a heavy mat. With the legs thus secured, the hands interlocked behind the neck, the body face down, you should lift your head and upper body off the floor as far as you can, then lower it; repeat the movement continually. An effective variation of this exercise is done by securing the upper part of your body and lifting both your legs simultaneously.

Other exercises which strengthen the lower back region include working out with a medicine ball, bending from the waist and touching the floor and various running and jumping exercises.

5. Special Exercises for the Feet and Legs

While your ability to use your feet and legs in jumping, walking and running depends to some extent on your over-all weight and the relative proportion of your trunk to your legs, the amount of spring in your legs depends very much on the condition of the muscles in your feet and legs. Some people retain great strength in their legs well into their fifties, while most others allow their condition to decline very sharply after they reach the age of thirty. According to an old saying among athletes, "It's the legs that go first," and while it is probably true that professional ball-players and fighters are forced to retire when their legs don't have it any more, the average person doesn't have to feel the adverse effects of weakening leg muscles, providing he keeps up a minimum of exercise.

The following exercises are especially recommended for people with low arches, pronation (the tendency to carry the weight on the inside rather than the outside of the feet), poor toe strength in jumping, walking and running, and poor leg and foot strength in hopping, vertical jumping, broad jumping, high jumping and running.

I. TOE PUSH–UPS

See Progressive Course, Lesson Two, Exercise IV b, page 114.

II. WALKING ON OUTSIDE OF FEET

See Progressive Course, Lesson One, Exercise V d, page 109.

III. VERTICAL JUMPS

See Progressive Course, Lesson Two, Exercise IV f, page 115.

IV. TOE–HEEL PRANCE

See Progressive Course, Lesson Five, Exercise III b, page 122.

V. Walk on tiptoes, working up gradually from 50 to 200 yards.

VI. Skip rapidly, working up gradually from 50 to 200 yards.

VII. Hop on both feet simultaneously, working up gradually from 25 to 200 yards.

VIII. BROAD JUMPS

Starting position: Standing.

Movement: Run a sufficient distance to work up a comfortable speed, then jump as far as you can. Repeat successively 10 to 50 times, trying for maximum distance each time.

IX. ENDURANCE HOPPING

Do the following hops continuously:

a. Hops on both feet simultaneously, up to 200 times.

b. *Jumping Jacks,* up to 200 times.
See Progressive Course, Lesson One, Exercise II h, page 105.

c. Scissor hops, shifting feet, forward and backward, up to 200 times.

d. Hops on right foot, up to 50 times.

e. Hops on left foot, up to 50 times.

f. *Squat Jumps,* as long as possible.
See Progressive Course, Lesson Six, Exercise IV b, page 127.

X. UPHILL TREADMILL WALK (10 TO 30 MINUTES)

Set the treadmill at an 8.6 per cent grade and a speed of 3½ mph. If a treadmill is unavailable, walk uphill or up and down a flight of stairs.

6. *Special Exercises for the Upper Body, Shoulders and Neck*

The peculiar demands of modern urban living prevent the muscles of the upper body and shoulders from being challenged to develop sufficiently. Since it is not necessary to chop wood, carry water buckets, or handle heavy tools, we are a civilization of human beings inadequately developed from the waist up. Particular attention should be paid to exercises which will strengthen this area of the body.

The key muscles of the upper body are those which help to pull the arms downward (*pectoralis major, teres major,* and *latissimus dorsi*). These muscles, together with the shoulder retractor muscles (*rhomboidei*), play an important role in such activities as chinning, rope climbing, swimming and throwing. Other important muscles in this area are those which flex the arms (biceps) and those which extend the arms (triceps). In spite of the fact that all of these muscles are employed extensively in tennis, baseball, basketball and football, the outstanding defect found in the muscular development of college freshmen is weak arm and shoulder muscles.

The following exercises are recommended for building up strength in the upper body, shoulders and back:

I. PUSH–UPS

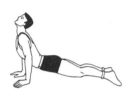

Starting position: Lying face down, toes inward so that insteps support feet; hands under shoulders and fingers pointed forward.

Movement: Easy Style: Lift your head first, then, as you straighten your arms, lift your chest, torso and legs in succession.

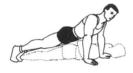

Intermediate Style: Straighten your arms completely, keeping your body straight and rigid throughout the press.

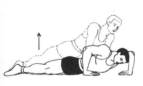

Hard Style: Move your hands farther out to either side of you, or move your hands out in front of your head, or turn your fingers in so that they point to each other, and press your body up, keeping it rigid all the time.
Repeat as many times as you can.

II. LEANING PUSH–UPS

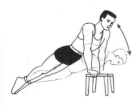

These are done the same way as intermediate push-ups, except at the starting position your hands and upper body should be resting on a low bench or a raised platform.

III. PULL–UPS

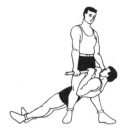

Easy Style: With heels resting on the floor, body rigid in a slanting position, and hands gripping a bar about 4 feet from the floor, with knuckles toward face, pull your upper body toward bar by flexing your arms until chin is touching the bar. Repeat as many times as possible. (The bar can be fixed across a doorway or can be a broom handle held by another person.)

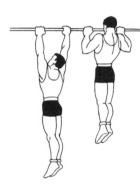

Intermediate Style: Hang straight from a chinning bar, with feet off the ground, and pull yourself up until your chin is over the bar.

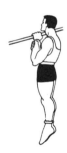

Hard Style: Grip the chinning bar with only one hand, place the other hand around the wrist of the hand holding bar, and pull yourself up until chin is over the bar. Repeat, using other arm.

IV. DUMBBELL EXERCISES

Use pair of 2-pound wooden dumbbells or 5-pound iron dumbbells.

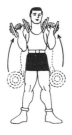

Curls: Assume a standing position, with arms hanging at sides. Flex your arms until dumbbells are shoulder high. Repeat 20 to 50 times.

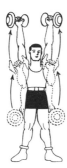

Curls Plus Overhead Press: Repeat curls. When dumbbells are shoulder high, press them overhead until your arms are fully extended above your head.

Chopping: Grasp one dumbbell in both hands and imitate motion of chopping with an axe.

Swinging: Holding a single dumbbell in one hand, swing your arm forward and backward, and then all the way overhead in a complete circle.

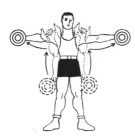

Four-count Exercise: (1) By flexing your arms, bring the dumbbells up to your chest; (2) extend your arms sideways until they are horizontal; (3) retract the bells to your chest; (4) lower the bells to your sides. Repeat 20 to 50 times.

V. MEDICINE BALL EXERCISES

a. Push pass to partner standing 8 to 10 feet away.
b. Overhead pass to partner standing 8 to 10 feet away.
c. With feet spread, underhand pass to partner standing 10 to 15 feet away.

    d. One-hand bowling style pass to partner standing 10 to 15 feet away. Alternate arms.

    e. Throw ball up against a wall from a lying position and from a standing position.

VI. PULLEY–WEIGHT EXERCISES

Starting position: Holding handles, with arms extended in front, standing far enough from pulley so that weights rest on floor but ropes are taut.

Movements:

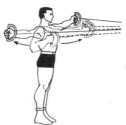

    a. Facing the weights, flex your arms, extend them to the side, return them to starting position.

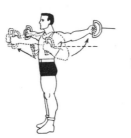

    b. Facing away from the weights, flex your arms, extend them to the side, and return them to starting position.

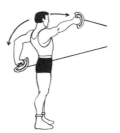

    c. Facing the weights, imitate swimming crawl stroke.

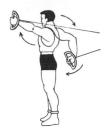

d. Facing away from the weights, imitate swimming back stroke.

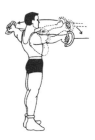

e. Facing the weights, imitate swimming breast stroke.

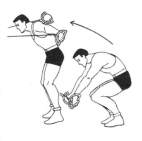

f. Facing the weights, imitate swimming butterfly stroke. See Progressive Lesson, Lesson One, Exercise II f, page 104.

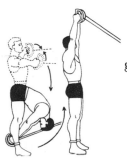

g. *Four-count rhythmic exercise:* Facing weights: (1) spread arms until they are fully extended sideways; (2) swing arms together and down, and pull between legs; (3) swing arms upward and extend overhead; and (4) return to starting position.

Index

interval training, 100, 142, 144
isometric exercises (*see* exercises, streamline programs of)

J

javelin, 43, 161, 167
jogging
between exercises, 111, 114, 134, 137, 139, 140, 149–150
during arm exercises, 109
in breathing and breath-holding exercises, 129
in Interval Training, 144
in place, 114, 149
in Relaxation Exercises, 157, 159
in Tapering-Off Exercises, 119, 146, 148, 150, 154, 157, 159, 160
in Warm-Up Exercises, 103, 111, 116, 121, 125, 129, 133, 142, 144, 151
on a treadmill, 161
to develop endurance, 85
Johns Hopkins University, 60
Johnson, Dr. Robert, 53
Jones, Dr. Hardin, 30
jumping
ability as an aspect of fitness, 41, 42, 43
Broad Jumps, 40, 47, 171
in exercises for feet and legs, 136
in exercises for the lower back, 170
in fitness tests, 39, 45, 47
Jumping Jacks, 105, 117, 159, 172
muscles used in, 42, 43, 170, 171
scissors jumps, 84
Squat Jumps, 63, 85, 89, 127, 128, 137, 154, 158, 161, 172
straddle jumps, 47, 84
Vertical Jumps, 115, 136, 137, 142, 171

K

kicking
Alternate Knee-Bend Kicks, 106, 111
between exercises, 111, 156
Flutter Kicks, on Back, 83, 147, 150, 153
Flutter Kicks, on Front, 107, 118, 130, 138, 143, 147, 150, 152, 153, 169
in Relaxation Exercises, 157
in Tapering-Off Exercises, 146, 148, 150
in Warm-Up Exercises, 111
muscles used in, 43
Scissors Kick, 167
Side Leg-Kicks, 106, 118, 123, 128, 150, 152, 154, 168
Sitting Frog Kicks, 149
skip-kicks, 108, 112
knees
Quarter Knee Bends, 114
Kolehmainen, Hannes, 92

L

latissimus dorsi, 172
legs
Alternate-Side Leg Lifts, 135, 138, 141, 143, 145, 158, 168
Alternate Single-Leg Lifts, 111, 122
exercises for, 74–75, 84–85, 89, 102, 108–109, 114–115, 122–123, 128, 133, 136, 139–140, 142, 143–144, 146, 163, 170–172
exercises for lateral muscles of, 73, 83, 88
exercises for leg extensors, 74–75, 84–85, 89
exercises for upper legs, 71–72, 82, 87
flexing, 67

ABOUT THE AUTHOR

Thomas Kirk Cureton, Jr. (Ph.D., Columbia University, 1939) is Professor of Physical Education at the University of Illinois, where he organized and has directed the Physical Fitness Research Center since 1944. The author of numerous books and texts, and some four hundred articles, he is widely recognized both in the United States and abroad as an authority on the scientific aspects of physical education and physical fitness research.

After studying the physical fitness of Army and Navy groups during World War II, Dr. Cureton developed objective methods for testing motor fitness, appraising human physique and some aspects of cardiovascular fitness. A Fellow of the American Association for the Advancement of Science, he was given the Roberts-Gulick Award for distinguished leadership in YMCAs of the United States, and in 1945 was elected Honorary Lifetime Fellow of the American Association for Health, Physical Education and Recreation. In 1947 he was elected a full member of the American Physiological Society, and subsequently became an associate member of the American Psychological Association and a member of the Royal Society of Health in England. He is also a Founding Fellow of the American College of Sport Medicine and has served on many committees of this organization.

Dr. Cureton's extensive activities include membership in the Physical Research Committee of the United States Army Air Force, and in the Joint Committee of the Federal Security Agency and the American Medical Association on Physical Fitness. He has also been a Consultant on Physical Fitness to President Eisenhower's, President Kennedy's and President

Johnson's Youth Fitness Council. He has served on the National A.A.U. and Olympic Committee for Swimming, and on the Medical and Nursing division of the Olympic Committee.

Dr. Cureton has given leadership to more than three hundred Physical Fitness Clinics in the United States and is internationally prominent as a teacher, researcher and lecturer in his field, having toured twenty-six countries in the interest of physical fitness work. His Illinois program has been featured on a coast-to-coast television program, "The Search for Human Health and Fitness."